WOMEN AND THE OWNERSHIP OF PMS

SOCIAL PROBLEMS AND SOCIAL ISSUES

An Aldine de Gruyter Series of Texts and Monographs

SERIES EDITOR

Joel Best

Southern Illinois University at Carbondale

WOMEN AND THE OWNERSHIP OF PMS

The Structuring of a Psychiatric Disorder

Anne E. Figert

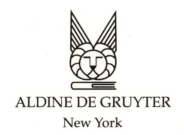

ALDINE DE GRUYTER

New York

About the Author

Anne E. Figert is Assistant Professor of Sociology at Loyola University, Chicago. Dr. Figert received her Ph.D. from Indiana University at Bloomington. She is the author of publications on the relationship of science and sociology as well as women and health.

Copyright © 1996 Walter de Gruyter, Inc., New York

ALDINE DE GRUYTER
A division of Walter de Gruyter, Inc.
200 Saw Mill River Road
Hawthorne, New York 10532

This publication is printed on acid free paper ∞

Library of Congress Cataloging-in-Publication Data
Figert, Anne E.
    Women and the ownership of PMS : the structuring of a psychiatric disorder / Anne E. Figert.
        p.   cm. — (Social problems and social issues)
    Includes bibliographical references and index.
    ISBN 0-202-30550-3 (alk. paper) — ISBN 0-202-30551-1 (pbk. :
alk. paper)
    1. Premenstrual syndrome—Psychological aspects.   2. Premenstrual syndrome—Social aspects.   3. Diagnostic and statistical manual of mental disorders.   4. Women—Mental health.   I. Title.   II. Series.
RG165.F526   1996
618.1'72—dc20   96-3647
                                                                      CIP

Manufactured in the United States of America

10 9 8 7 6 5 4 3 2 1

For my grandmother Ruth Hunt,
and my mother Elaine Figert

Contents

PART II   THE THREE DOMAINS OF CONFLICT

Acknowledgments

There are many people who deserve and need to be publicly thanked for their efforts in helping this book along its way. First of all, I have been fortunate to meet many of the people involved in the LLPDD controversy. Their willingness to talk to me and share their feelings about the events surrounding the inclusion of LLPDD in DSM-III-R impressed me and spurred me to produce this work. I also had the good fortune to initially work with four outstanding scholars. Professor Thomas Gieryn of Indiana University is my mentor and trusted advisor. For his encouragement, challenges and support, I will always be grateful. Bernice Pescosolido has also been a key person in shaping my life and professional world. I learned a great deal about medical sociology and the professions from Bernice. Donna Eder and Ellen Dwyer are my feminist inspirations. I learned about gender scholarship from both of them.

I received financial support for the initial research in the form of a fellowship from the Indiana University Graduate School. Their research grant made my archival trips to Washington, D.C. possible. Dr. Roger Brown of the American Medical Association helped me with library access and retrieval of some important sources of information. Jackie Hickey worked with me to initially conceptualize the figures in Chapter 4. The Center for Instructional Design at Loyola provided further assistance. Joel Best, the editor of this series, also helped me tremendously with his comments on earlier drafts. At Aldine de Gruyter, Richard Koffler and Arlene Perazzini shepherded me through the publishing process with great care, skill and humor. I appreciated that very much. Mr. William Baxter, former Librarian and Archivist of the APA Library, was also extremely helpful and patient. Finding the time to write this book was harder than I thought it would be. I received a semester leave of absence from Loyola University Chicago to conduct further research on this topic. The APA's kind permission to make use of the Diagnostic Criteria for the LLPD is gratefully acknowledged.

My colleagues in the Department of Sociology and Anthropology at Loyola University Chicago have been especially kind and patient with me. In particular, Mark Shibley, Fred Kniss, Kathleen Adams, Peter Whalley, and Judy Wittner proved to be life savers and read many drafts of the chapters. The graduate students at Loyola have also had to endure my use of

xi

LLPDD as an example in many courses and in thinking about their own work. In particular, I would like to thank Reid Helford, Colleen Carpenter, Lynn Higgins, Todd Campbell for listening or reading parts of the manuscript. Karen Chase and Vanessa Reichartinger provided essential computer support during the last days of manuscript preparation.

I am also grateful for the permission granted to use the cartoons and various PMS exhibits in Chapter 1. Thanks to Patricia Kadel, Steve Phillips and Creatif Licensing Corp. of Mount Kisco, New York, Leslie Murray and Design, Inc. of Grand Rapids, Michigan, and Audrey Christie and Recycled Paper Products, Inc. of Chicago, Illinois. An addition thanks to Kay Turner and Girls in the Nose Productions (P.O. Box 49828 in Austin, Texas 78765) for the use of the lyrics from "Menstrual Hut." Portions of Chapter 4 were adapted from "The Three Faces of PMS: The Professional, Gendered and Scientific Structuring of a Psychiatric Disorder," copyright 1995 by the Society for the Study of Social Problems. Reprinted from *Social Problems*, vol. 42, No. 1, February 1995, pp. 56–73.

Finally, I owe a profound debt to my family and friends. My family instilled me with a love for learning and supported me through many years of education. Eric Wright provided me with ice cream, books and tracked down key references at the last minute. Heidi Mason, Starla Sholl, Lisa Frohman and Nancy Mathews supplied friendship and good conversation. Finally, Jeanne Kerl lived through the entire project and made constructive comments. Her historian's insight and demand for detail has made this book a better product. Her love and support have made me a better person.

Glossary of Terms and Organizations

APA The American Psychiatric Association. Founded in 1844, the APA has approximately 34,000 members and an annual budget around $20,000,000. It publishes the DSM.

Apa or APA The other APA; the American Psychological Association. It opposed the inclusion of a PMS-related diagnosis in the DSM-III-R and DSM-IV.

DSM The basic reference book for the mental health field. It provides standardized diagnostic criteria for mental health workers and insurance carriers. Seen as representing the American Psychiatric Association's and psychiatric profession's consensus on the diagnoses of mental disorders.

DSM-III-R Revised edition of DSM-III published in 1987.

DSM-IV Revision of the DSM-III-R published in 1994.

ICD International Classification of Disease is a statistical classification of diseases by the World Health Organization (WHO). As a statistical classification the ICD indicates the relationship between diagnostic categories and is *not* a nomenclature, i.e., a list or catalogue of approved terms for describing and recording clinical and pathological observations.

ICD-9-CM Developed for use in the United States in 1978 to provide clinical and technical guidance to clinicians and patient care-givers. Includes all of the final DSM-III and DSM-III-R classifications.

LLPDD Late Luteal Phase Dysphoric Disorder. Diagnosis placed in the Appendix of the DSM-III-R. Originally called premenstrual dysphoric disorder (PDD), then periluteal phase dysphoric disorder (PPDD).

Designed as a subset of PMS conditions in which mood disturbance is a predominant symptom.

PMDD   Premenstrual Dysphoric Disorder is in the main text of the DSM-IV as an example of a depressive disorder. The research criteria remain in an appendix of DSM-IV.

PMS   A term for which there is no precise definition.

Introduction

Is Premenstrual Syndrome a mental illness? On June 23, 1986, after a year of bitter dispute, the Board of Trustees of the American Psychiatric Association said yes and placed a premenstrually-related diagnosis in an appendix—instead of the main text—of the soon to be published revised third edition of its *Diagnostic and Statistical Manual of Mental Disorders* (DSM-III-R). The psychiatric manifestations of PMS became something called Late Luteal Phase Dysphoric Disorder (LLPDD). Since 1994, LLPDD has been known as Premenstrual Dysphoric Disorder (PMDD) and is listed in the main text of the DSM's fourth edition, DSM-IV. So, the short answer to the question is yes, a form of PMS is an official mental disorder. It is official because the DSM is seen as a basic reference book for all mental health professionals. It provides standardized diagnostic criteria used by most insurance carriers and is recognized by the federal government and the courts as the psychiatric profession's consensus over the diagnoses of mental disorders.

LLPDD was originally proposed under the name Premenstrual Dysphoric Disorder (PDD) in June 1985 by an advisory committee to the American Psychiatric Association (APA), composed of scientific and medical experts on premenstrual syndrome. They hoped that it would isolate severe psychological and emotional symptoms found in a small percentage of women during the premenstrual phase. This advisory panel, later called the LLPDD Advisory Committee, defined and established the parameters of the diagnosis, and voted to recommend inclusion of PDD in the DSM-III-R. But these deliberations—on their surface an obvious case of scientific consensus over a proposed diagnosis—quickly erupted into a major public problem.

A campaign organized by women psychiatrists and mental health professionals to stop the inclusion of this and two other controversial diagnoses was soon underway. The primary charge by the opposition was that the diagnosis would be stigmatizing to all women. Letters and calls of protest soon flooded the offices of Robert Spitzer (the Chair of the Work Group to Revise the DSM-III) and the American Psychiatric Association. Articles appeared in newspapers, magazines, and newsletters. The opponents met with a newly appointed Ad Hoc Committee to evaluate the revision process of the DSM, and held a public protest at the Annual APA meeting in Washington, D.C. In short, the inclusion of the PMS-related diagnosis became a public controversy.

THE OWNERSHIP OF PMS

The decision to include LLPDD in the DSM-III-R was so controversial and consequential, because it concerned many people—not just women and psychiatrists—who were trying to define and claim "ownership" of PMS. Gusfield defines the "the ownership" of a social problem in the following way:

> To 'own' a social problem is to possess the authority to name a condition a 'problem' and to suggest what might be done about it. It is the power to influence the marshalling of public facilities—laws, enforcement abilities, opinion, goods and services—to help resolve the problem. (Gusfield 1989:6)

In linking Gusfield's term of ownership with PMS, I argue that LLPDD was not just an issue for the two opposing groups, but for a constellation of often overlapping actors and social groups. All were trying to claim ownership of PMS and its psychiatric manifestation in LLPDD. The decision to place LLPDD in the appendix of DSM-III-R was the result of the conflict and interests in three domains of interaction: The health and mental health domain, the woman domain, and the science domain. These domains (Chapters 5, 6, and 7) were shaped and formed by various players in the controversy—health care professionals, feminists, women with PMS, journalists, gynecological researchers, and many more—whose different beliefs and values, goals, and interests also shaped what became LLPDD into not one but multiple, distinctive phenomena.

To understand how and why the inclusion of LLPDD was so controversial, Chapter 1 examines Western cultural images of women with PMS and their role in setting the climate for the LLPDD controversy. For example, jokes, cartoons, and over-the-counter medications all depict an image of a "crazy" woman at the mercy of "her raging hormones." In Chapter 2, I argue that the inclusion of LLPDD was also consistent with epistemological and organizational changes occurring in the profession of psychiatry in the latter twentieth century. Public perceptions of the field of psychiatry and the American Psychiatric Association were important as the controversy over LLPDD was interpreted from a variety of different perspectives. To get a clear picture of what really happened in the LLPDD/DSM-III-R controversy, I construct a straightforward narrative account in Chapter 3.

Chapter 4 sets the stage for the questions and analyses that are addressed in the rest of the book: How was the controversy portrayed or explained in public accounts? How do multiple sources of power and interest shape scientific truth and bureaucratic decision-making? How did these multiple actors claim "ownership" of PMS in the LLPDD controversy? Three different public accounts of the controversy emerged: an economic account, a political account, and a rational account. Economic accounts portrayed the inclusion of LLPDD as a result of economic expansion by psychiatrists and the APA. Political accounts made the eventual decision to include LLPDD in DSM-III-R into a matter of competing professional and gendered powers and interests, and centered attention on "obviously political" actors (e.g., "feminists" and "psychiatrists"). Rational accounts make the decision into a matter of science (evidence and logic) and bureaucratic procedure (rational and formal) within the American Psychiatric Association. I argue that the economic, politics, and rationalities surrounding the construction of LLPDD did not come together in one way but in three—depending upon the chosen domain of analysis. LLPDD took on multiple realities during the debate and controversy of its construction. I describe a domain analysis and the three domains and ownership claims from which LLPDD emerged.

In Chapter 5, I examine LLPDD from the first of the analytical domains: the health and mental health domain. Drawing on sociological works on the professions and especially psychiatry, I develop LLPDD as an artifact over which gynecologists, psychiatrists, psychologists, psychiatric nurses, and social workers all struggled for control. I contend that in this domain, LLPDD involved a battle for professional dominance, and justify that conclusion in part through empirical analysis of participants' actions and interpretations as the diagnosis came into being.

In Chapter 6, LLPDD becomes a different object, one embedded in struggles for control over the definition of a "normal and healthy woman." It is the ubiquitous "woman's" body and mind that are being contested. Historical associations of menstruation and madness are explored, centering on the particular case of premenstrual syndrome. In the woman domain, feminist health, mental health, and political groups/individuals engaged in a gendered struggle against the effect of the diagnosis LLPDD labeling all menstruating women as potentially "crazy." Steps taken by professional women to prevent inclusion of LLPDD consisted of coalition building, holding meetings and protests, and initiating a letter writing campaign. Individual women with PMS also enter this domain of analysis by claiming that their condition is biological, not psychiatric. Other professional women fought to include LLPDD in the DSM on the grounds that it would help individual women suffering from PMS. In this domain, then, LLPDD becomes a "label" to be promoted or opposed and a legitimate description of some women's experiences in the premenstrual phase of their menstrual cycle. In the same way, when situated in feminist theories and critiques of science, gender studies, and historical and anthropological studies of women and menstruation, LLPDD becomes a gendered artifact related to issues of stigmatization and control of women's bodies.

Finally, in the science domain (Chapter 7), LLPDD is either a scientific fact that represents the natural world, or scientists' social construction of a reality that exists only through their forces of persuasion. Both sides of this argument are represented in the battle to define and control the scientific "truth" about PMS and LLPDD. When controversies rooted in scientific or medical "facts" go public—and competing versions of the truth enter the fracas—the image of science as a politically neutral and disengaged authority may be at risk. How these controversies get settled often depends on how and when the rhetoric and authority of science are used to bolster some claims while undercutting others. Based upon the belief that "the truth WILL out," the APA Board of Trustees voted in the end to place LLPDD in an appendix—in effect, calling for and further justifying the need for more scientific research. LLPDD becomes both "fact" (something real) and "artifact" (something made) when situated in the literature from sociology, history, and philosophy of science and technology.

The costs and benefits of a three-domain analysis in the study of a scientific controversy are explored in my conclusions (Chapter 8). I suggest that an answer to the question "Who won the battle over LLPDD?" depends on which domain one enters and, thus, on which reconstruction of events one prefers. The analysis ends with some reflections on a sociological methodology that does not seek the one best explanation. What is gained by using literatures from sociology—not as mere tools for analysis, but as part of the phenomenon itself—are further resources through which LLPDD gets constituted.

Finally, I conclude this study by showing in the Afterword (Chapter 9) how and why the APA changed LLPDD back into Premenstrual Dysphoric Disorder (now called PMDD) and included it in the main text of the manual's 1994 edition (DSM-IV). New actors, changing interests, and old arguments are presented in documenting the latest installment in the PMS/DSM drama.

MY DATA COLLECTION EXPERIENCE (AND FASCINATION) WITH THIS TOPIC

When I first heard about the possible inclusion of a PMS-related diagnosis in the DSM-III-R, I was certain that I had found the perfect case study. Here was a clear case of how the predominately male psychiatric profession was putting the proverbial screws to women. Or was it? Everything that I read initially about the controversy indicated that here was a case where "feminists" were battling psychiatrists over the authority to define the parameters of a mentally healthy woman in modern society (see more about this in Chapter 5). It was—and still is—an engrossing controversy and people were—and still are—fascinated by the idea that PMS could be classified as a psychiatric disorder.

With all the certainty and zeal of the beginning stage of any research project, I set out to document how the scientific and medical professions were making antifeminist and antiwomen statements by placing LLPDD in the DSM-III-R. What I discovered was that it is not quite that simple. In this study, I utilized primary data from several sources. I conducted semi-structured personal interviews with four key participants, two proinclusion (Robert Spitzer and Sally Severino) and two anti-inclusion (Jean Hamilton and Teresa Bernardez) psychiatrists who took public stances and played a leadership role during the controversy.

I also examined the APA archival records and materials deposited at the American Psychiatric Association headquarters in Washington, D.C. These records consisted of internal memos concerning the DSM-III-R and LLPDD, letters of protest written about LLPDD, and minutes of meetings of committees involved in the DSM revision and the LLPDD decision. To balance the official records and documents of the APA, I also gained access to the bulk of the anti-inclusion materials that are deposited at the Institute for Research on Women's Health (Washington, D.C.). These records consist of briefing and press booklets, petitions, and strategic correspondence about fighting the inclusion of LLPDD.

Finally, I collected and examined published accounts of the controversy in the popular, medical, and scientific presses. Any reference or mention of the DSM-III-R or LLPDD was counted as data for this study. The data in this study—articles, interviews, written documents (letters, memos, diagnoses)—are all texts of some form. From a methodological and analytical point of view, this is a study of texts within various social, political, and professional contexts. The multifaceted data collection methods allowed me to understand how LLPDD was constructed through negotiation, debate, and contestation over time. By focusing upon the content and nature of these different texts, my analysis differs from traditional discourse analysis because I treat discourse as data (a resource) and not as the subject (a topic) of study. The discourse in all of these texts became the means or resource for analysis and not an end or object of analysis in itself.

But I also ran into some issues that I had not counted on or thought about. Let me describe three important events for you:

1. When she heard what I was writing about, a friend's grandmother told me that she favored the inclusion of LLPDD in the DSM-III-R because she thought that it would prove that what she felt as a

young woman was "real," even though nobody would believe her at the time. I was reminded in a very personal way that this was a "real" issue in women's lives—that some women do feel validated by the official nature of the inclusion in the DSM. This helped me gain understanding about the nature and effect of this controversy on individual women's lives.

2. During my interview with him, Robert Spitzer (one of the psychiatrists interviewed for this study and head of the DSM-III-R Work Group) asked me if I was a feminist. When I replied yes, he then asked me whether my own personal politics would allow an accurate analysis of this controversy. At the time, I was put off by his question. However, I am now glad that he challenged me because I actively and consciously worked to ensure that all sides and perspectives in this controversy were heard.

3. I had the opposite experience when I interviewed the two psychiatrists who were against the inclusion of LLPDD. Because I am a woman, a sociologist, and am interested in this topic, I think that it was taken for granted that my ideas and politics about the inclusion of LLPDD mirrored theirs. Interest in this subject could come only from a sympathetic ally—which was and remains true. It would have been very easy to write this book from the perspective of someone who is totally opposed to making PMS a psychiatric disorder.

Throughout the research and writing process, I was constantly reminded about the effect of something called PMS in women's lives or asked to state my position on PMS. I was just trying to be a good sociologist and figure out what happened and make sense of it. My training in the sociology of scientific knowledge insists that "things are not always what they appear." In scientific controversies, there are multiple positions and interests, and these could change over time. Sociologists are trained to be critical and skeptical even though they may personally believe in something as "real" or "wrong." So, as I investigated this controversy and began to analyze the data that I collected, I tried to keep an open mind about the people, events, and results that took place during the LLPDD controversy.

The result is my attempt to analyze the LLPDD controversy from a sociological perspective and to suggest this perspective produces a much more complicated picture than the "official," personal, or media accounts. I do not believe that there are any "right" and "wrong" sides in this controversy—just complicated issues, scientific and political stances, and, most of all, people—from the anonymous woman with PMS, to the scientists and mental health professionals, to anti-inclusion protestors at the APA convention in 1985. This book is about **all** of the people, events, and issues involved in this controversy.

Setting the Stage

1

Is PMS Real?:
PMS as Scientific and Cultural Artifact

Is PMS "real"? If the APA's *Diagnostic and Statistical Manual of Mental Disorders* includes a PMS-related diagnosis, then are all or most premenstrual women mentally ill? These are questions that I am often asked. I am not always sure how to reply. I think that most people who ask these questions (usually women) want a medical opinion or validation that I am not comfortable (or qualified) to give. In my mind, any answers to these questions are political answers. My usual answers are yes, PMS is real; and no, all menstruating women are not mentally ill. The longer version of my answer implies that there are many variations and versions of what and how something is "real." An old axiom in sociology (paraphrased and based upon work by W.I. and Dorothy Swaine Thomas) suggests that if people define things as real, then they are real in their consequences (1928:572).

In this chapter, I show how PMS is real because various people in different situations choose to define it as such. For example, when I first started investigating this topic in 1989, I clipped a three-sentence news item from the local newspaper, the Bloomington (IN) *Herald-Telephone*. The headline read: "School may change its PMS initials," and the item began: "Officials are considering changing the name of Pendelton Middle School or at least removing its initials from athletic uniforms to avoid embarrassment for its girls' teams." When and why did the initials PMS become such a source of embarrassment that people would actually consider changing a school's name or buying new uniforms? Who was more embarrassed? School officials or the girl's athletic teams? I never found out, but I knew that I had to understand the history and cultural meanings attached to PMS in my attempt to understand why LLPDD was so controversial. So, my question was, how is PMS "real" and why?

In this chapter I explore the various definitions: PMS as a medical condition, as a social scientific and feminist issue, as an explanation for women's behavior and moods in the popular culture, and, finally, as something bought or sold in a market. The first answer to these questions takes

3

us into the realm of science and medicine and how PMS came to be a twentieth-century (and particularly) Western notion of a treatable disease. A second set of explanations comes mostly from academic studies of how menstruation and PMS are firmly rooted in cultural notions and ideas about women and their role in society. A third way to explain PMS explores how its shape and image construct women's bodies and minds in western popular culture. Part of the force behind this cultural portrayal of women and PMS comes from a fourth way in which PMS obtains definition—the PMS industry, which has tried to shape and explain PMS in a certain way (as something that makes women "crazy" and uncomfortable) to sell products.

What does this discussion have to do with whether or not premenstrual women are mentally ill? The image of women and how PMS is defined sets the stage for the discussion of how and why the American Psychiatric Association began to consider the inclusion of a PMS-related diagnosis in the DSM. Each of the ways that defines PMS as real helped to define the debate and controversy over whether PMS (as defined in LLPDD) is a psychiatric disorder. The discussion that follows does not attempt to provide the reader with a cultural history of PMS. There are several good articles and books that do this (Golub 1992; Delaney et al. 1988; Martin 1987; Buckley and Gottlieb 1988). However, it is important to provide evidence for my argument that PMS has become an important part of current Western culture and society's definition of women.

THE SCIENCE OF PMS

The primary way in which new ideas or diseases achieve legitimacy or recognition in modern society is for scientists or physicians to call them real. Scientists and physicians have the "cognitive authority" in society to "define, describe or explain bounded realms of reality" (Gieryn and Figert 1986; see also Starr 1982 for a discussion of "cultural authority"). When M.D.s or Ph.D.s in chemistry or biology believe something is real, people usually go along with them. This is what happened to PMS in its various forms and incarnations in the twentieth century: PMS became real as a medical diagnosis and condition.

American gynecologist Robert Frank was the first to publish scientific studies about a condition he called "premenstrual tension" (1931). Frank identified excess estrogen as the cause of observed symptoms of this "medical" condition, which he described as hormonal in origin:

These patients complain of unrest, irritability, 'like jumping out of their skin' and a desire to find relief by foolish and ill considered actions. Their personal suffering is intense and manifests itself in many reckless and sometimes reprehensible actions. Not only do they realize their own suffering, but they feel conscience-stricken toward their husbands and families, knowing well that they are unbearable in their attitude and reactions. Within an hour or two after the onset of the menstrual flow complete relief from both physical and mental tension occurs. (1931:1054)

What is more interesting in this article are his published comments about particular case studies. Under a list of patient complaints, Frank's notations include "husband to be pitied," "psychoneurotic," "suicidal desire," and "sexual tension" (Frank 1931:1055). Frank's prescription for severe cases of premenstrual tension was either complete removal of or radiation therapy ("X-ray 'toning'") upon the ovaries to decrease estrogen production in the body and thus to restore order in both the home and the workplace.

Between 1931 and 1980 there were steady references to premenstrual issues in the medical literature. In her review of the PMS literature, Rittenhouse states: "[a]uthors generally constructed PMS as a medical phenomenon requiring management and treatment by a physician or a psychiatrist/psychologist. However, PMS was not seen as a major problem for the majority of women" (Rittenhouse 1991:416). Nor was PMS seen as a *major* research problem for most scientists.

PMS as a medical disorder received steady but relatively little attention until an English doctor, Katharina Dalton, began to investigate it. In 1953, Dalton co-authored an important article on PMS in the *British Medical Journal* (Greene and Dalton 1953). This article first introduced the term "Premenstrual Syndrome," emphasizing that women need not accept the physical and emotional discomfort of PMS every month, and that modern medicine could help them.

Dalton has conducted research and written articles and books on PMS for over 40 years. She defines PMS as "any symptoms or complaints which regularly come just before or during early menstruation but are absent at other times of the cycle. It is the absence of symptoms after menstruation which is so important in this definition" (1983:12). According to Dalton's research, PMS is responsible for decreased worker productivity (in both the sufferer and "her husband"), increased divorce rates, and even murder. Dalton presents cases for her theory using vignettes of PMS sufferers and displays of medical/biological charts of women's hormonal cycles. She continues to argue for the medical control of women's hormones through progesterone therapy, prescribed by general practitioners and assisted by psychiatrists and gynecologists (1983:191).[1]

Dalton's own popularity, notoriety, and authority as a PMS "expert" heightened when she served as the chief defense medical expert in a 1981 murder trial in London, in which she successfully argued that the defendant was not responsible for murdering her lover because she suffered from a severe form of PMS (see Laws et al. 1985 for an account of this trial). The publicity generated from this trial and Dalton's claims of successful progesterone treatments found many different audiences in the United States and brought publicity to PMS.

Due in part to the publicity generated by these trials, PMS and related diagnoses have been called the "disease of the 1980s." As one science writer stated, PMS had "arrived." A disease that thousands of women had been told did not exist suddenly become a media event (Heneson 1984:67). More importantly, Heneson points out that PMS acquired medical legitimacy: "After years of telling women their problems were 'all in the head,' the proportion of doctors who accepted PMS as a real disease reached critical mass" (1984:67).

A specifically bio-medical orientation to PMS defines it as a medical problem requiring a specific type of scientific research, diagnosis, and intervention. Scientific research has been conducted on premenstrual issues since the 1930s and the term "premenstrual syndrome" was coined in 1953. The result is that PMS is real in the scientific and medical sense. As explored further in Chapter 7, the way that PMS was constructed as a medical artifact and public interest in the 1980s strongly influenced the exploration and development of what became LLPDD.

PMS AS A FEMINIST SCIENTIFIC ARTIFACT

Feminist writers are quick to assert that the very use of the term "premenstrual syndrome" is an attempt by scientists to make premenstrual "tension" a more scientific term, and takes the control of women's bodies out of their own hands (Laws et al. 1985:17). The use of the word "syndrome" instead of "symptoms" itself suggests that there is an underlying disease process in women's bodies (Ussher 1989:73).

Ironically, it was feminist researchers (especially in nursing and psychology) who were responsible for conducting a significant portion of the scientific research done on PMS during the 1970s and 1980s. Since the 1970s, feminist scientists have actively worked within the field of science to study PMS and to make sure that the research was conducted. Feminist critics of menstrual and premenstrual studies have long argued for different and better scientific methodologies, more appropriate research designs, and nonstigmatizing labels and assumptions (Koeske 1983). So, feminist scientists took responsibility for the majority of scientific research on menstruation in the 1970s and 1980s because they believed otherwise it would not be conducted (Parlee 1992; Tavris 1992). For example, professor

Alice Dan states that she helped found the Society for Menstrual Cycle Research in 1979 to fill in the "gaps" left by scientific research and its distortion of women's experiences (Dan and Lewis 1992). Fausto-Sterling identifies researchers such as Parlee, Dan, Koeske, and Golub as "a new wave" of menstrual-cycle scientists who have a "full respect for women" and do not reduce "human behavior to some simple biological variable" (1985:108). Feminist scholars "had to press for research funds and scientific attention to be given to a bodily process that only women experience. Many women themselves have responded positively to the language of PMS, feeling validated at last by the attention being paid to menstrual changes" (Tavris 1992:133).

In the eyes of many early feminist researchers, PMS was initially a "woman's topic" and, therefore, not considered an important area of research for mainstream scientists and medical researchers. Psychiatrist Jean Hamilton (who was actively involved in fighting the inclusion of LLPDD) believes that another reason why PMS research was done primarily by women was that male researchers did not take seriously studies of menstruation and menstrual disorders: "It's funny because I think originally some women were doing research on the menstrual cycles, particularly women in psychology, were doing it primarily because, I mean, no man was going to do it. It was neglected" (personal interview, Jean Hamilton, June 1990).

Another PMS scientist (Parlee) states that this research by feminist scientists also had a political purpose:

> In the early and mid '70s some social scientists, mostly feminist psychologists, began focusing on menstruation as a 'new' research topic, one about which academic psychology had been silent for more than 25 years. They did this in response to an antifeminist political rhetoric in the public domain which argued that social relations of gender in the family and workplace . . . are justified by objective scientific facts about women's bodies and minds. Psychologists took this rhetoric at face value as being about science and scientific truth, and sought to contest claims about 'raging hormonal influences' within the scientific domain with logical reasoning and empirical data. (Parlee 1992a)

Thus, these early feminist researchers sought to "demystify" the negative stereotypical images of women and PMS by conducting "good" and "sound" science.

So, what scientifically constitutes PMS—and how PMS research should be legitimately carried out—were questions raised by feminists within the scientific profession in the 1970s and 1980s. The aim (and possibly its result as well) of feminist scientific work on menstruation was to refute negative images of PMS using the tools and rhetoric of science. These feminists

believed that changes in public perception and attitudes about the previously understudied topic of menstruation and PMS were achievable from
within science.

SCHOLARLY AND SOCIAL SCIENCE EXPLANATIONS
OF PMS/MENSTRUATION

While physicians and scientists studied and tried to define PMS and other menstrual disorders in terms of biology, mainly feminist anthropologists, sociologists, and other scholars tried to place and account for PMS in
its social and cultural context. The second wave of feminism in the 1960s
and 1970s was the impetus not only for studying PMS scientifically but for
studying how PMS was portrayed as debilitating to women's bodies and
minds. Studies of the history of menstruation in human society point out
that menstrually related disorders are often associated with the practice of
labeling women and their behaviors crazy (dating back to ancient Greek
writings) (see Delaney et al. 1988; Martin 1987; Olesen and Woods 1986).
Scholars have linked PMS to ancient descriptions of hysteria and other
modern characteristics (lethargy, moodiness, and depression) previously
attached to menstruation itself (Gottlieb 1988; Rodin 1992).

For example, in some cultures, menstruation has been portrayed as an
evil spirit that invades women of childbearing age once a month (for reviews of this historical association see Weideger 1976; Delaney et al. 1988;
and Fausto-Sterling 1985). Cultural taboos and negative stereotypes—such
as not touching a menstruating woman and physically separating her—
have also existed. For example, in their book *The Curse*, Delaney et al. point
out:

> Eskimo believe that contact with a menstruating woman can lead to bad luck
> in hunting; the contamination takes the form of an invisible vapor which at-
> taches itself to the hunter so that he is more visible to game and therefore un-
> able to catch it. Among the Habbe of the western Sudan, a man whose wife
> is menstruating does not undertake any hunting. Bukka women may not go
> into the sea to bathe for fear of spoiling the fishing. (1988:10–11)

The Ancient Greeks believed that "the wanderings of the uterus in
women's bodies were thought to cause all sorts of unusual behaviors—behaviors that bear a striking resemblance to those attributed to PMS today"
(Rodin 1992:50).

Other authors have tried to combat negative stereotypes of madness-
and-PMS by tracing the diagnosis (as a cultural and political artifact) to
capitalist patriarchal society. Martin argues that PMS is historically locat-

ed within the stresses of modern capitalism in western culture (1987). For Martin, PMS is a natural site for rebellion by women due to their oppressed situation, but that science and industry have colluded in subverting menstruation and generating the need for artificial hormone and psychiatric treatment of women. Martin asks how is it that "a clear majority of all women are afflicted with a physically abnormal hormonal cycle"? (1987: 114). Her answer is that it is no accident that the initial interest in what is now called PMS emerged during the 1930s: "It strikes me as exceedingly significant that Frank was writing immediately after the Depression, at a time when the gains women had made in the paid labor market because of World War I were slipping away. Pressure was placed on women from many sides to give up waged work and allow men to take the jobs" (1987:118).

Katharina Dalton's and other post-World War II studies that emerged in the 1950s also appear to fit into this pattern of medical claims to diagnose and treat problems in the home and workplace. These medical studies have a distinct focus on the effect of a woman's PMS on her social roles of wife, mother, and worker. As Bell (1987) points out, this early scientific work on PMS stressed how disruptive it is in the home, factory, and social order. By focusing on this "disruption," Bell is able to show how the medical community has attempted to claim ownership over PMS and to medicalize women's bodies:

> This perspective assumes that 'normal' families are happy and that women are responsible for preserving happiness of the individual family members. In this respect, the medical literature attributes problems in families (unhappiness, arguments, and violence) to women in general and PMS in particular, and recommends that they can be solved medically. This locates the problems and solutions within the family. A specific individual—the woman—is then identified as the source of her behavior. This kind of reasoning mitigates against the possibility of exploring men's contributions or other social roots and social solutions to these problems. (1987:167)

Another author identifies the specifically male composition of the medical profession as the source of control and power over women's bodies and PMS. In the introduction to *Seeing Red: The Politics of Pre-Menstrual Tension*, Jackson writes that women need to "suspect that the possibility of diagnosing PMT [PMS] increases the power of the medical profession over our minds and bodies, enabling them to redefine real conflicts and tensions in our lives as sickness, and put pressure on us to conform" (as quoted in Laws et al. 1985:7).

Other feminist writers and health care providers have tried to communicate the need for every woman to take control over her body and its byproducts, such as menstruation and PMS (Rome 1983). In a recent article in *Ms.* magazine, members of the Boston Women's Health Book Collective continue their advocacy by claiming that "the cure for PMS may lie in resocialization and societal change, not medicine" (1992b:76). Other examples of more "popular" health care explorations of PMS include pamphlets by the National Women's Health Network and a plethora of recent books on PMS and menstruation (explored later in this chapter).

Sociologists and anthropologists have suggested that in fact PMS is a "culture bound syndrome." Johnson states that it

> involves bizarre behavior which is recognized, defined, and treated as a specific syndrome only by biomedical healers in Western, industrial cultures, and can be only understood in this specific cultural context. (1987:347)

Johnson argues that in western culture PMS serves as a symbolic mechanism for both the structural maintenance of society and for its social change due to the role conflict in which women find themselves. In this role conflict, women are expected to be productive (have a job/career outside the home) and to be reproductive (to have a family/children). Thus, PMS simultaneously and symbolically denies the possibility of each because "in menstruating, one is potentially fertile but obviously nonpregnant; in having incapacitating symptomatology one is exempted from normal work role expectations. With PMS, women can be seen as 'victims' who did not 'choose' to be sick" (Johnson 1987:349).

This theme of role strain/conflict among western women is echoed by Pugliesi (1992), who proposes that "what is labeled as PMS is actually deviation from normative expectations regarding emotion" (1992:132). The pressure on a woman to "have it all" (career and family) gets symbolically released once a month in her PMS. Rodin explains how the PMS category and its explanation are consistent with western cultural themes about women's reproductive systems, "abnormal behaviors," and the gendered roles of wife and mother (1992:50). Gottlieb takes "as a given" that PMS fits into late industrial society in the ways described above. Yet, she believes that women's subversion of "normally expected" gendered traits during the premenstrual time (and calling this PMS) is ultimately harmful because it allows people (including the woman herself) to trivialize and dismiss these feelings and anger (1988).

The social, scientific, and feminist analyses in this section suggest that the diversity of meanings assigned to PMS in contemporary Western culture (e.g., bitchy, moody, not responsible for behaviors, and uncontrolled emotional states) is related to the societies in which they are developed and is also indicative of the movement in modern society to assign a medical label or explanation for human behaviors.

POPULAR IMAGES OF WOMEN, MENSTRUATION, AND PMS

PMS also has a very real image in the popular culture of something that drives women crazy once a month. Both women and men have tried to explain women's unusual behaviors or bad moods as the result of the impending occurrence of the "monthly visitor." How PMS is portrayed and used in everyday life is yet another aspect of how PMS is real. I have a collection of PMS "artifacts" that I have been accumulating over the years. Friends and colleagues have provided me with a wide range of PMS jokes, anecdotes, shirts, buttons, and coffee cups. If (as the section above argues) PMS is firmly ensconced in modern, western industrialized society and its values, what exactly does this image consist of?

I looked to my PMS archive to see how women and PMS fit together and tried to find some common themes. These themes are at the same time shocking and funny *or* not shocking and not funny. What did I find? A wide variety of images of women as subject to their raging hormones, engaging in "abnormal" behaviors, and jokes that portray women as "bitchy," "mean," and "illogical." On the other hand, I also found images of women that were powerful and that try to "harness the energy" of PMS.

The most commonly cited example of cultural attitudes about PMS is the "Woman in Authority with Raging Hormones scenarios." We can probably trace the "raging hormones" idea to a public statement by Edgar Berman, Hubert Humphrey's physician during the 1968 Presidential campaign. Berman stated that he did not want a woman in a position of power because she would be subject to "raging hormonal influences" each month (as cited in Corea 1985; Fausto-Sterling 1985). Berman clarified his views on the subject in a 1976 interview with journalist Gena Corea: "'Menstruation may very well affect the ability of these women to hold certain jobs,' he told me. 'Take a woman surgeon. If she had premenstrual tension—and people with this frequently wind up in a psychiatrist's office—I wouldn't want her operating on me'" (as quoted in Corea 1985: 106–107).

Even Hollywood romances are not safe from PMS attacks. *People* magazine reported in 1994 that when Melanie Griffith filed for divorce from Don Johnson (and then withdrew the petition a day later) that it was "an impulsive act that occurred during a moment of frustration and anger" and attributed to Griffith's PMS. According to the article, Griffith "told an interviewer, 'I have terrible PMS, so I just went a little crazy'" (March 28, 1994:43). Griffith later divorced Johnson (for reasons presumably other than PMS), but the PMS-made-me-crazy excuse offered a convenient account for what was seen at the time as an "impulsive" or "crazy" action. This negative image of women is also evident in the jokes, greeting cards,

television shows, and even the advertisements for over-the-counter medications for PMS (Chrisler and Levy 1990; Pugliesi 1992).

The most common site for this attribution of "women subject to their
raging hormones" is PMS humor. PMS jokes or humor themes have become common on television and in movies, often used as interpretations
of women's "abnormal" or "deviant" behavior. A couple of years ago, an
episode of the popular show *Roseanne* depicted a day in the life of the entire family affected by Roseanne's (the wife and mother) rapid mood
swings, emotional outbursts, and unpredictable behaviors. Even an
American icon of womanhood is not immune to PMS. Patricia Kadel's
"PMS Barbi" is tragically transformed and warns the reader "Don't toy
with me!"

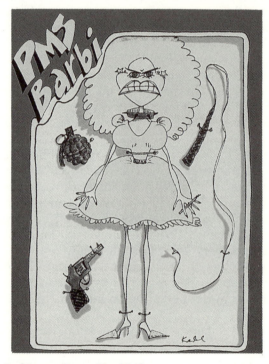

Illustration 1.1.   Barbi transformed by PMS.
    From "PMS Barbi" West Graphics, Copyright © 1992 Patricia Kadel. Reprint-
    ed with permission.

Some jokes about PMS have been particularly vicious. The following
joke appeared in the 1980s during the time in which pit bulls became popular as attack dogs and there were numerous public reports of these ani-
mals mauling young children: "What is the difference between a pit bull

and a woman with PMS?" The answer to this question is that "A pit bull doesn't wear lipstick." Another joke appeared during the Gulf War crisis in 1989–1990: "Did you hear that they pulled 15,000 soldiers out of Saudi Arabia? They replaced them with 5,000 women with PMS because they're three times meaner and they retain water better." PMS also has its own "screw in a light bulb" joke contained in the following greeting card: Why does it take three women with PMS to change a light bulb? Answer: It just does!!

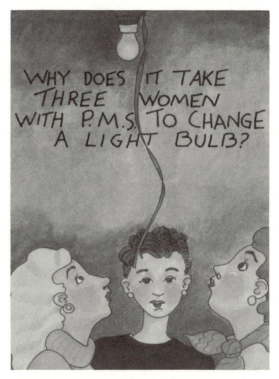

Illustration 1.2. PMS stereotypes in a common joke formula.
From © Recycled Paper Greetings, Inc. All rights reserved. Original design by Audrey Christie (Steve Philips). Reprinted by permission.

I have two different versions of greeting cards to send people with this joke: What is the difference between a woman with PMS and a terrorist? Answer: You can negotiate with a terrorist. My favorite graphic version of this joke looks like this:

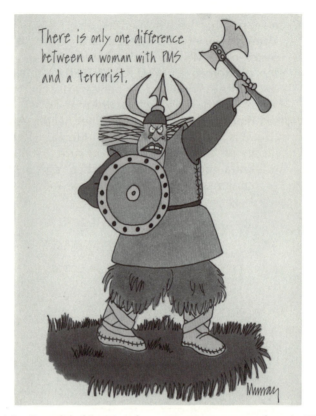

Illustration 1.3. Images of irrational women are commonplace in PMS humor. From: *Reason with a terrorist* © 1991 Design Design Inc. Artist/author Leslie Murray. Reprinted with permission.

I also have a button that warns the reader: "I've got PMS. Stay the Hell Away!" On the other hand, my coffee cup queries: "I've got PMS. What's Your Excuse?" This suggestion that somehow women might be excused from their normal roles and sanity during the premenstrual phase is taken even further in a humor book about PMS called *Raging Hormones: The Unofficial PMS Survival Guide*. The authors define a "hormone hostage" as "Any Woman who for Two to Fourteen Days Each Month Becomes a Prisoner of Her Own 'Raging Hormones' and Plummets Her Life and the Lives of Those Around Her into an Unholy Premenstrual Netherworld" (Williamson and Sheets 1989:10). This book goes on to describe and portray various ways in which "hormone hostages" act and are affected by PMS such as "Do's and Don'ts of the Premenstrual Workplace," "How to Tell PMS From Your Own Stupid Character Flaws Quiz," and "The PMS-Elvis Connection."

One of the most popular and influential PMS cartoonists is Steve Phillips. He has drawn a variety of PMS postcards, calendars, and greeting cards. His series of "PMS Attacks in Literature" include a Juliet screaming "Romeo, oh Romeo . . . WHERE THE HELL ARE YA!!" and a very bloated Snow White surrounded by her dwarfs. His "PMS Attacks in History" characters include a crying Joan of Arc and a Marie Antoinette that was so bloated that she could not quite fit her head through the hole of the guillotine. But it is Phillips's contemporary female character Melinda who faces a variety of "PMS attacks" at work and at home. In the following cartoon, Melinda goes a little crazy in her "spring cleaning" by throwing and destroying major appliances, clothes, and other household fixtures.

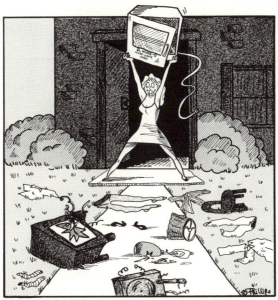

To take her mind off her PMS, Melinda decides to do a little spring cleaning

Illustration 1.4. Another image linking irrationality with a woman's PMS. From: PMS attack, 1990 calendar, 1989 publication. Copyright © Steve Philips.

In PMS Attack #2, Melinda is faced with an unpleasant realization that her life is similar to a spin-cycle of a washer and bursts into tears. The punch line of this greeting card states that "Life's a bleach and then you dye."

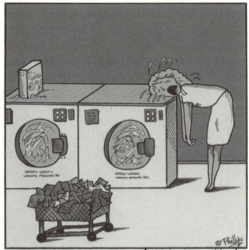

While at the Laundramat, Melinda suddenly
bursts into tears as she realizes the
similarities between the spin-cycle and her life

Illustration 1.5. PMS humor often equates the symptoms of PMS with sudden
mood swings.
From: Copyright © Recycled Paper Products, Inc. Original design by Steve
Philips. Reprinted with permission.

Melinda's life and her PMS attacks often reflect the previously discussed
scholarship on the relationship between role/gender conflict and modern
society. Melinda falls asleep at work during an important meeting; she sits
at her desk wanting to kill everyone in sight; she impulsively hacks off
most of her hair. In a series of cartoons, Melinda's PMS affects her relationship with her boyfriend Barney in a variety of ways. In one cartoon,
Barney arrives for his date with Melinda in a full suit of armor; in another,
he looks uncomfortable when she starts crying in the middle of a movie;
and finally Barney is scared (mouth and eyes wide open) when Melinda
drives the car in an erratic manner "to take her mind off her PMS."

PMS humor has also gone "high tech." I recently found a PMS Cartoon
Gallery on the internet at a World Wide Web site on women's health created by a physician. Mark Perloe states:

> PMS is a serious problem that can be debilitating for those suffering from its
> effects. The loss of control, mood swings and depression often impairs one's
> function within the family and at work. The cartoons displayed here are not
> meant to offend, or belittle the seriousness of the problems PMS sufferers
> have to face. Humor can often serve as an introduction to discuss a sensitive

subject. That is the sole purpose wherein this material is provided. (1995:http://www.mindspring.com/~mperloe)

Perloe's introduction to his PMS gallery suggests an important point with which I found myself struggling. At what point does PMS humor belittle or harm women with PMS and at what point is something "funny"? This is something that I became aware of as I analyzed my PMS artifact collection. The images and humor are contradictory and ambivalent. Granted some of the jokes (e.g., the pit bull joke) are in bad taste and do promote an extremely negative image of women. On the other hand, "PMS Barbi" seems like a perfect and ironic inversion of the stereotype of the perfect American woman.

Laws makes a similar point in her study of British men's attitudes toward menstruation. As schoolboys, their use of humor to talk about menstruation was different than the way in which schoolgirls used slang and made jokes about their periods. While growing up, boy's humor was more derogatory, and usually contained sexual references and a way to 'get at girls.' But, Laws points out the dilemma: "I certainly do not want to imply that taking an entirely solemn attitude to periods would do girls any good. Laughing at one's own bodily functions and the inconveniences they bring with them is a healthy sign and is quite different from the 'them and us' joking of the boys" (Laws 1990:72). The authors of *Hormone Hostage* take on their critics in their Authors' Note:

> Some will say that a humorous book about PMS will set women back a hundred years. We say that no one can ever move forward without confronting and controlling the obstacles that threaten to impede her progress.
> And, we say that sometimes the best way to start taking something seriously is with a sense of humor. We may mock the syndrome and its symptoms, but never the women who struggle with them. (Williamson and Sheets 1989)

Humor and other popular images of women and PMS that appear on the surface to promote a negative image of women might instead also be suggesting alternative (and even positive) images for women. For example, an alternative rock band from Austin, Texas called *Girls in the Nose* have a song called "Menstrual Hut" on their album (Girls in the Nose 1987). This song starts out with the following words:

> I'm bleeding down below
> I'm bleeding from my brain
> My hormones kick in
> They're driving me insane.
> (Words by K. Turner, Copyright 1987 by Peterson/Turner)
> Band: Girls in the Nose. Reprinted with permission)

However, this song goes on to explain that modern science and medicine will not in help in women's experiences with the menstrual cycle. What is really needed is the return to a menstrual hut (used in other cultures) and its monthly release from traditional women's roles of cooking, cleaning, and family duties. This thought is echoed in a cartoon that I recently saw that portrayed an obviously worn out woman holding a screaming child and telling her husband (sitting in a lounge chair and reading the paper) that "this is stress, not PMS."

Other attempts to subvert the dominant thinking and image of women in PMS is contained in a favorite button and expression around my house: "PMS—Harness the Energy." Another expression found on a t-shirt defines PMS as: Putting Up with Men's Shit! Dena Taylor wrote *Red Flower: Rethinking Menstruation* (1988) as a response to women's negative comments about menstruation and as a vehicle to elicit more positive associations among women. The book contains poetry, stories, and other positive expressions about PMS and the menstrual cycle. The author states: "My goal is to show that women do celebrate and honor menstruation. I want to help dispel the idea that menstruation is shameful, that it should be kept hidden. We need to recognize this part of our cycle—to be aware of its subtle and powerful effects on us, and to see these in a way that enriches our lives" (Taylor 1988:1). This book is consistent with other attempts such as the song "Menstrual Hut" to elucidate the overlooked positive changes that occur with women's menstrual cycle such as vivid dreams, more creativity, and energy.

How does this conflicting image of women and PMS (as both negative and positive) in the popular culture address the question of whether or not PMS is real? I think that it does more to solidify the image of women being ruled by their hormones. For better or worse, women's actions, moods, and feelings are being portrayed (by men and ourselves) as subject to influence of their menstrual cycle. This cycle "makes" them "go crazy," "be bitchy," and "be irresponsible." Furthermore, this excuse is seen as "legitimate" because it is based upon scientific and medical research. Since PMS seems to change women's moods and mental state, one next logical step would be to legitimate PMS as a psychiatric disorder.

THE PMS INDUSTRY

The discussion of PMS humor and artifacts brings us to the important consideration that one very significant way in PMS is "real"—that PMS is an industry. The PMS industry consists of what I call the 3 P's (products, pills, and prescriptions). Most of the PMS humor and artifacts are found as products that are bought and sold in the economic marketplace. The postcards, greeting cards, calendars, cartoon and humor books, and songs all come with a price tag attached. Greeting cards currently cost anywhere from $1.25 to $3.00; books, calendars, and t-shirts run in the $10 to $15 range. PMS products will be available as long as people are buying these and other PMS-related products.

Another set of PMS products are pills. In her examination of the creation and proliferation of PMS as a disorder, Eagan argues that there is a strong connection to the drug companies and treatment options (Eagan 1983). The drive for profits by drug companies exploits women:

> Often when a drug suddenly makes the news, or when a new 'disease,' for which there is a patented cure is discovered, it is fairly easy to find the public relations work of the drug manufacturers behind the story. (Eagan 1983:81)

Over-the-counter remedies for PMS symptoms are available at local drugstores or through the mail for those times when you cannot "control the witch in you" (Heneson and Strain 1984). For those women that can afford it, more sophisticated hormone and antibiotic treatments are available at specialized PMS clinics or from your family physician to "tame the shrew in you" (Lehrman 1988; Payer and Gross 1989; Sneed and McIlhaney 1989).

In the early 1980s, the pharmaceutical industry began to offer specific over-the-counter PMS drugs and more PMS-related products (Willis 1983). According to a cover story in *Drug Topics* on menstrual products:

> Much of the growth of menstrual pain relievers could be traced to the premenstrual syndrome segment. While PMS products accounted for only 5% of total menstrual pain reliever sales in 1983, they moved up to 20% in 1984. (Ehrlich 1985:45)

A marketing consultant quoted in the same article attributed this surge in PMS over-the-counter products both to manufacturers' marketing of new products and to increased media attention of PMS. He stated that "[b]oth have raised women's awareness of the need to take a PMS product in addition to taking a product during menstruation" (as quoted in Ehrlich 1985:45).

The market for over-the-counter PMS products was so great that the Food and Drug Administration (FDA) came up with its own definition of PMS in 1982. Its Advisory Review Panel on Miscellaneous Over the Counter Internal Drug Products defined PMS as

> A recurrent symptom complex that begins during the week prior to menstruation and usually disappears soon after the onset of the menstrual flow. This symptom complex consists predominantly of edema, lower abdominal

pain (including cramps), breast tenderness, headache, abdominal bloating, fatigue, and the feelings of depression, irritability, tension and anxiety. (as quoted in Golub 1992:182)

In 1983, this Advisory Review Panel released a review of over-the-counter PMS products. The panel recommended that various combinations of analgesics, diuretics, and antihistamines be considered effective PMS products (see Willis 1983 for a full report). They maintained that analgesics provide relief for pain, cramping, and headaches; diuretics give the relief of water retention and bloating; and antihistamines relieve a variety of symptoms such as depression, irritability, weight gain, swelling, and backache. These over-the-counter treatments are considered safe and effective for mild to moderate symptoms of PMS.

But over-the-counter PMS pharmaceuticals were not the only product benefitting from increased attention to PMS in the early 1980s. A third part of the PMS industry is the prescriptive part. PMS treatment centers using progesterone therapy (that Katharina Dalton advocates) also became popular during the early 1980s:

Progesterone's first big boost in America as a treatment for PMS came with the establishment in 1981 of the National Center for Premenstrual Syndrome and Menstrual Distress. Despite the imposing name, the 'national center' was actually established as a privately owned, profit-making clinic. The Manhattan office (there was also one in Boston) charged $165 for three visits, plus another $50 to $100 for lab costs. (Heneson 1984:68)

One gynecologist worried that such clinics would attract women who are desperate for help—ones who "can be easily ripped off. They're paying $5 for a 50-cent product [progesterone suppositories]. They're being told they're crazy, so they'll do anything" (as quoted in Heneson 1984:69). According to this doctor, science and "legitimately" approved pharmaceuticals—not "rip-off" progesterone clinics—provided better, safer, and cheaper treatments for women with PMS.

Another important piece of the PMS industry is the PMS self-help books. Most of these books are soft cover, relatively inexpensive ($3–7), have been written since 1980, and are found in mainstream bookstores. Most of these books are written (solely or in joint authorship) by physicians or therapists associated with PMS or Women's Health clinics (e.g., Lark 1984; Norris and Sullivan 1983; Nazzaro and Lombard 1985). They usually include short histories about PMS, and medical, nutritional, and exercise advice to overcome its symptoms.

So, according to the pharmaceutical industry, government officials, women with PMS, or authors of books, the key to defining PMS was as something that can be helped with pills, diets, and other products offered in the PMS industry. Thus, PMS is very real—complete with price tag attached to it.

WHAT'S AT STAKE IN THE CONSTRUCTION OF PMS?

For some women, the publicity and legitimization of PMS and its symptoms as real, a natural part of their body and its processes, have led to a positive sense of control over this phenomenon. However, a more negative image of PMS as something that controls women once a month, that makes them "crazy" and subject to their hormones, is much more pervasive in our contemporary Western culture. This image has allowed women to use PMS as an excuse to express their emotions or to account for their otherwise "strange" behaviors. Other people (husbands, children, doctors, lawyers, judges, juries, co-workers) have also used PMS to explain women's behaviors—often within a scientific or medical framework that then gives physicians and scientists "expert" legitimacy over women's bodies and minds. PMS has been tried as a legal "insanity" defense in cases involving women accused of murder or other crimes in the United States, but with little success.[2] A recent book by Caplan (1995) reports cases in which the threat of using PMS in child custody cases kept women in abusive relationships. In addition, a well-publicized case involved a female physician who successfully used PMS to get off of a drunk driving charge in 1991 (*Washington Post* Editorial June 8, 1991:A20).

How PMS is defined—and who controls or owns the diagnoses related to it—has been and continues to be a matter of social, political, and economic concern. The degree to which "PMS" has become a major issue is best understood in light of current estimates that anywhere between 20 and 90% of all women would qualify as having some of the more than 150 recognized symptoms of PMS (Olesen and Woods 1986; Adler 1990a). According to the American College of Obstetricians and Gynecologists, it is normal for women to experience some premenstrual symptoms. This organization more conservatively estimates that some 20 to 40% of all menstruating women do experience some symptoms of PMS (see Adler,1990a). These changes include physical symptoms such as weight gain, bloating, and aches of all kinds, as well as emotional symptoms such as irritability, mood changes, and even positive symptoms such as vivid dream cycles.

As I have shown in this chapter, PMS has been defined in a variety of ways (scientific, feminist, cultural, and economic) over the years, but there is no consistent or agreed upon definition. If the estimates given above are indeed true, and if almost all menstruating women do have at least some of these symptoms, then the "stability" of women's moods and behaviors can be called into question by scientists, doctors, politicians, bosses, and lawyers. This directly links to the issue of the inclusion of a PMS-related diagnosis in the DSM. What is considered "normal" for women itself is at the heart of the debate in the PMS/LLPDD controversy.

NOTES

1.   The FDA does not approve of progesterone for the treatment of PMS, and there have been no scientifically proven studies documenting the efficacy of progesterone treatments.

2.   The so-called PMS defense is most successfully used in England and in France. It has not had such success in American courts (Benedek 1988; see also Chaite 1986 and Allen 1990).

2

Setting the Stage:
The DSM and the American Psychiatric Association

> There is something solid, permanent, and official about a list of symptoms in a scholarly-looking tome like the *Diagnostic and Statistical Manual of Mental Disorders*. The DSM is the mental equivalent of the *Physician's Desk Reference*, the medical dictionary all doctors rely on. (Tavris, *The Mismeasure of Woman* 1992:177)

To understand the story of LLPDD, we cannot begin in 1985 when it was first proposed for inclusion in the DSM-III-R. We need first to understand what the DSM is, what it represents, and why it is important to study; second, we need to understand the role of the DSM in the larger organizational context of the American Psychiatric Association. As the quotation by Tavris indicates, the DSM is, first, a book. It looks, and is, very official. The DSM-III-R (the edition that included LLPDD) has over 500 pages of charts, tables, diagnoses, and definitions of mental disorders. The DSM is also much more than a book; it is also a system for classifying and diagnosing what is officially recognized as a mental disorder.

Today, if you complain of "feeling down" or "upset," your doctor may pull out her DSM-IV to see if you qualify for the diagnosis of "depression, not otherwise specified." This diagnosis will determine whether she prescribes certain drugs or therapies for you and whether this visit will be covered by federal government health programs or your insurance company. For example, if you are a young woman and complain of being depressed or moody due to PMS, you may be given the diagnosis of premenstrual dysphoric disorder and a prescription of Prozac (an expensive antidepressant). From 1987 to 1994, you may have been given the earlier diagnosis of LLPDD. Prior to that, you were on your own to convince the doctor that something was indeed "wrong" with you. In seeking treatment, you have to weigh the issue of being labeled or diagnosed as having a mental disorder in order to have your condition and prescription covered by your in-

surance policy. What do you decide? Do you risk being labeled as mentally ill and having this on your medical chart? How will this diagnosis of
having a mental disorder affect the rest of your life? Will prospective em-
ployers, friends, or lovers look down upon you? Will this label be used
against you in child custody proceedings in which your mental stability is
called into question?

The DSM, which is owned, published, and controlled by the APA, has a
major influence on the lives and legal rights of everyday citizens. It dictates
the way in which mental disorders are defined, shaped, and formed and
has very real consequences in people's lives. Take another example—this
time a case in which a specific disorder was taken out of the DSM. Prior to
1983 and the publication of the DSM-III, gays and lesbians were officially
defined as mentally ill—not just for same-sex behaviors but for their feelings (see Bayer 1987 for a detailed study of this). Millions of people were
defined in this century as "sick" for something that most people understand today as human diversity in sexuality. People were often hospital-
ized and treated without their consent (with electroshock, drugs, and even
surgery) because parents, judges, or physicians were able to point to the
DSM definition of homosexuality as a mental disorder. Although a form of
homosexuality (ego-dystonic homosexuality) was listed in the DSM-III,
the category has been eliminated since the publication of the DSM-III-R in
1987. The ramifications of this decision to eliminate homosexuality from
the DSM have been enormous. Today, gays and lesbians no longer have to
fight the official medical label of being mentally disordered and have used
the elimination of the diagnosis from the DSM to fight for larger political
and social acceptance in society.

What is, or is not, in the DSM as an "official" mental disorder matters.
Each edition of the DSM serves as the psychiatric profession's current consensus over mental disorders. The inclusion of the diagnosis LLPDD was
controversial in part because, like other issues of mental health, it involved
a debate about the source of individual people's problems. The central issue in any debate about mental health is the location of a person's mental
distress. Is this distress a biological *disease* and therefore mental *illness?* Is
this distress wholly rooted in the societal pressures, where certain behaviors are labeled as inappropriate? Or is it a combination of both biological
and social forces that combine to influence a person's thinking and behavior? These questions revolve around the so-called nature vs. nurture debate about human behavior. It also points to reasons for what might have
appeared, on the surface, to be an attempt to increase scientific knowledge
about the connection between women's bodies and their moods, but, instead, erupted intò a major public controversy. I argue in this chapter that
the development of the DSM in the twentieth century also requires an understanding of the formation and history of the American Psychiatric As-

sociation in 1844. The intersection of history and organization of the APA influenced the development of the DSM and, ultimately, of LLPDD.

THE AMERICAN PSYCHIATRIC ASSOCIATION

What began as a correspondence between two superintendents of hospitals for the insane to discuss mutual problems in caring for this unique population of patients eventually led to the establishment of the organization that would become the American Psychiatric Association. In 1844, Thomas S. Kirkbride, superintendent of the Pennsylvania Hospital for the Insane, invited all other superintendents of hospitals for the insane to meet in Philadelphia to discuss their mutually unique problems and possible solutions (McGovern 1985). "The Association of Medical Superintendents of American Institutions for the Insane" was founded as a result of this initial meeting. It was the first organization of medical professionals in the United States, preceding the American Medical Association by 3 years. As the name of this organization indicates, psychiatry and the Association were closely tied to the mental asylum (Grob 1983).

The profession of psychiatry "grew from a more diffuse humanitarian concern, combined with a view of environmental causation [of mental disorders]" (Neff et al. 1987:50). Solutions included standards for the location, design, and construction of mental hospitals (issued in 1851), and a "moral treatment" of the mentally ill, which included loosening the restraints and occupational therapy (Baxter and Hathcox 1994). The basis of "moral treatment" meant that

> [t]he sick person had to be hospitalized in order to remove him or her from an environment that doctors believed had been both the precipitating and a contributing cause of insanity. In the hospital the doctors' individual attention, firm but kind treatment, and reluctance to use physical or mechanical restraint gained the confidence of the patient. Doctors then put into effect a program that interjected stability into the patient's life by its very regularity. Each asylum had a daily schedule of rising, eating, exercising, and socializing that varied only according to summer or winter hours. (McGovern 1985:10)

The institutionalization of moral treatment plans and the meetings with other hospital superintendents constituted a concerted effort to professionalize the medical care of persons with mental problems. In fact, historians point out that the founding members of the psychiatric profession deliberately tried to distance themselves in the public eye from the general medical profession. At the same time, they were also trying to indicate and claim their own expertise as medical specialists dealing with the mentally ill (McGovern 1985; Grob 1983, 1994).

By the end of the nineteenth century, however, many psychiatrists shifted their private and public affiliation from custodial care, and began to identify more closely with the medical specialty of neurology (Grob 1994). Psychiatry as a profession was undergoing considerable conflict in its professional identity and affiliation. Neurologists looked to the causes of insanity in the brain and central nervous system. For psychiatrists, this meant that if insanity was rooted in the body, then behavioral reform efforts in the asylum would not, in principle, work. In trying to align and reintegrate the profession back into modern medicine, psychiatrists began to look for scientific investigations into the causes of mental diseases and for data on how to treat severe illnesses and not just provide custodial care for their patients.

These shifts in ways of thinking about and doing psychiatry were so primary to the professional thinking about their mission that they changed the name of their professional organization—twice. The public name changes—in 1892, the Association of Medical Superintendents of American Institutions for the Insane became the American Medico-Psychological Association, which, in 1921, became the American Psychiatric Association—meant that certain intellectual segments of the profession had enough power and control to alter the professional image of psychiatry. How a profession names itself and presents itself to the public is important. As Bucher and Strauss indicate:

> Those who control the professional associations also control the organs of public relations. They take on the role of spokesmen to the public, interpreting the position of the profession, as they see it. They also negotiate with relevant special publics. (1961:332)

The early twentieth-century practitioners created a new psychiatry—one that "was fundamentally transformed from a discipline concerned primarily with insanity to one equally concerned with normality, as focused on normal persons and their problems as on the recognized insane" (Lunbeck 1994:3). Lunbeck argues that as psychiatry moved away from the institutional arrangements of the custodial care of the "insane," a new form of thinking took hold. No longer was a dichotomous classification of sane versus insane sufficient. The concept of normality became a continuum of a person's behaviors and symptoms and their fit to the environment. Grob (1994) further describes this shift as a move to "dynamic psychiatry" as psychiatry moved out of the mental asylum and into the larger community.

The advent of World War II marked another major shift in the profession of psychiatry. The armed services initially used psychiatrists to weed out draftees who had or might experience mental problems in the ranks. However, there were not enough trained psychiatrists to accomplish this task and it did not work very well. Psychiatrists and other physicians were not very successful in predicting who might have problems in battle situations. The result of this failed attempt in the armed services and psychiatrists' treatments of soldiers in wartime had profound implications for the profession of psychiatry and its knowledge base. According to Grob, psychiatry reevaluated itself once more and came to the conclusion that (1) mental disorders were far more common and serious than thought, (2) environmental stress plays a major role in mental problems, and (3) early treatment in noninstitutional settings could produce favorable results (Grob 1994:91). The major epistemological implication was that psychiatric interventions in community and family settings might be more effective than institutionalization of the mentally ill.

It was also at this time that psychodynamic and psychoanalytic psychiatrists were taking positions of leadership within the APA and on medical school faculties (Grob 1991). The rise of treatment protocols such as electroshock therapy, lobotomies, and psychotropic pharmaceuticals (such as thorazine) also helped reduce a postwar image of psychiatry working outside the walls of the insane asylum, in the larger community. More importantly, none of these treatments required a precise psychiatric diagnosis. Thus, psychiatry was once again in the position of redefining its relationship with the rest of the medical profession. In the aftermath of World War II, federal funds were allocated for psychiatric services and the training of psychiatric professionals—through the Veteran's Administration and the passage of the National Mental Health Act in 1946 (Grob 1994). This act established the National Institute of Mental Health (NIMH) within the division of the National Institutes of Health (NIH). This identification of NIMH within NIH was important, because it further served to identify mental health within biomedicine and to provide for the research and training of a whole new generation of psychiatrists and social scientists interested in mental health and illness. So, at the same time that research funds were available to study mental health and illness and effective medical treatments were established, the leadership of the APA took a psychodynamic approach, which viewed the person's mental health problems as more than just a medical problem.

Harvey Smith, a sociologist writing in the 1950s, offered the following explanation for the medical–biological shift in psychiatry:

> Psychiatry has shifted its scientific base away from medically respectable neurology and has moved toward a psychodynamic orientation. These psychodynamics have often found little support within the medical profession, and have been freely used by lay therapists. This provides a dilemma for psychiatry—the very sources of its medical distinction are often only marginally acceptable to medicine. Some physicians, including psychiatrists, lump

the non-neurological aspects of psychiatry with the social sciences and reject them accordingly. (1954:312)

Smith convincingly shows that while psychiatry was an outsider in medicine, it was very much an insider among other mental health professions: "[i]n this area of overlap psychiatry, the medical *outsider*, plays the powerful role of a *medical* speciality in confronting nonmedical groups. Its status, and the power of organized medicine, may operate to effect the continued subordination of nonmedical psychotherapeutic groups" (1954:315).

The insider/outsider dance of ambiguity with the rest of the medical profession continued to affect the profession of psychiatry in the last half of the twentieth century. In the past 30 years, American psychiatry went away from the psychodynamic approach and has taken on a more medical emphasis in diagnoses and treatment of mental disorders. A recent editorial in *The Lancet* locates the conflict for the profession in the question: "Is psychiatry really about disorders of the mind or disorders of the brain" (1994:681). In defense of this resurgence of the biological and medical models, some psychiatrists argue that it is merely the result of a need for further systematization and legitimization of psychiatric research (Klerman 1977; Blashfield 1984). Critics have argued that the recent shift to biomedicine and this "decade of the brain" is a conscious professional effort on behalf of psychiatrists to control the mental health hierarchy of labor (Kirk and Kutchins 1992).

I argue that the relationship of psychiatry with the medical profession and medical model is best explained by locating it within two phenomenon: first (1) pressure to label and diagnose mental disorders—which led to changes and developments of the DSM; and (2) the APA's response by social critics about labeling and the antipsychiatry movement.

PSYCHIATRIC NOSOLOGY AND THE DEVELOPMENT OF THE DSM

Throughout the twentieth century, American psychiatry did not have much interest in nosology or the classification of mental disorders.[1] The first system of classification was established in the United States in 1917 by the American Medico-Psychological Association—the result of a 3 year effort with the National Committee for Mental Hygiene. The title of this first effort was *The Statistical Manual for the Use of Hospitals for Mental Diseases*. It was published with the National Committee for Mental Hygiene.

According to Barton, the *Diagnostic and Statistical Manual of Mental Disorders* "emerged out of the perceived need for an official classification by military psychiatrists during WWII" (Barton 1987:282). At the end of World

War II, there were four major classification systems competing with each other: a standard system adopted by the APA in 1932, in U.S. Army classification, the U.S. Navy classification, and the Veteran's Administration system (Blashfield 1984). The standard classification used by the APA was deemed obsolete by military psychiatrists because it underrepresented less severe and psychosomatic disorders (Frances et al. 1994). Under the direction of the United States Public Health Service, a working group of psychiatrists designed a new nosological scheme adequate for the needs of modern psychiatry. It was also designed to be an alternative in the United States to the International Classification of Diseases (ICD-6) mental disorders section. In 1952 this working group published the DSM-I, which "represented a major effort on the part of American psychiatry to establish the boundaries of its work" (Bayer 1987:39). At the time of its publication, however, "psychiatric diagnosis was unpopular" due to the heavy influence of psychoanalysis in American psychiatry. Moreover, the DSM allowed only one diagnosis per patient, which some psychiatrists felt was limiting (Robins and Helzer 1986:410, 416).

The DSM has been revised four times. The DSM-I and DSM-II heavily mirrored the influence and popularity of psychoanalytic perspectives on mental health and disorders (Gaines 1992). The DSM-II was published in 1968, and was developed to be consistent with the mental disorder section of the eighth edition of the *International Classification of Diseases* (ICD-8), published by the World Health Organization. According to Blashfield, "The DSM-II represented the culmination of the movement to create a classification system that was a consensus of accepted concepts and that could be used for the purpose of communication" (1984:21).

DSM-III AND THE NEO-KRAEPELINIAN SHIFT

Psychiatry's recent turn toward classification and biological explanations of psychiatric disorders has been called the "neo-Kraepelinian" shift (for a description see Brown 1987, 1990 and Blashfield 1984). Emile Kraeplin was an early French psychiatrist interested in identifying and categorizing mental illnesses. The so-called "neo-Kraepelinians" of American psychiatry have "asserted the positive values of classification, advocated the medical model, and strongly favored a research approach to psychopathology based on genetics and biochemistry" (Blashfield 1984:35). This movement also contains psychiatrists "who oppose the psychoanalytic perspective, and who are very much interested in research" (Blashfield 1984:21). For example, a recent article by Mathis points out that the use of lithium in the early 1970s created a situation where the development of specific, precise psychiatric diagnoses was important for the successful treatment of patients. He states that the "[a]ccuracy of diagnosis became all-important to the psychiatrist treating a psychotic patient" (1992:255). The use of lithium as an effective treatment for manic depression reduced the number of people being diagnosed with schizophrenia and once again redirected the psychiatric profession's ties to the medical profession.

The rise of this school, and the declining influence of psychoanalytic thought, refocused psychiatrists thinking on diagnostic issues (Robins and Helzer 1986). Part of the neo-Kraepelinian focus is to systematize psychiatric diagnoses, and Robert Spitzer (the Head of the Work Group to Revise DSM-III and DSM-III-R) has been a part of this movement as a member of the "Washington—St. Louis Group" (see Blashfield 1984; Robins and Helzer 1986). Spitzer has stated his desire not to be considered a member of the neo-Kraepelinians but as a scientist who is concerned with empirical data issues (see Klerman 1986).[2] However, in spite of these denials, the DSM-III and DSM-III-R (whose changes were under the control of Spitzer) are generally portrayed and seen as the organizational and scientific achievement of the neo-Kraepelinian movement in psychiatry. Indeed, others have painted it as a complete paradigm shift in the field of psychiatry, which is exemplified in current editions of the DSM.

The DSM-III (published in 1980) represents the apex of the influence of this shift back to the importance of psychiatric diagnosis. According to Barton, these revisions prove that psychiatrists "have demonstrated the move from a symptom oriented typology toward a more etiological focus as scientific discovery permitted" (Barton 1987:280). In addition, Wilson establishes that more than just an epistemological change occurred with the DSM-III's publication. He states:

> The history of the development of the DSM-III is a story about the changing power base, as well as the changing knowledge base, within American psychiatry. Clinicians were replaced by biomedical investigators as the most influential voices in the field. (Wilson 1993:408)

THE RELATIONSHIP OF DSM-III AND DSM-III-R

The DSM-III-R was published in 1987. If the DSM-III was such an advancement in psychiatric nosology, why revise it so soon? According to the APA, revisions to DSM-III were necessary for a number of reasons. First, the APA has tried to make the DSM consistent with the mental disorder's section of the World Health Organization' (WHO) *International Classification of Diseases* (ICD). The United States has treaty obligations to make certain disease classifications compatible with the WHO's classification

system for worldwide comparisons. In 1976, the APA helped in the modi-
fication process of ICD-9 to facilitate use of this classification system in the
United States. The product, ICD-9-CM, made it possible for most of the developing DSM-III classifications and its diagnostic terms to be included in
the ICD-9-CM classification.

Because the ICD was not scheduled for revision until 1992, the APA Board
of Trustees decided that the span of time between the publication of DSM-
III (1980) and ICD-10, projected to occur between 1992 and 1994, was too long
a period to wait. The publication of DSM-IV was scheduled to coincide with
the 1993 publication of ICD-10. All of DSM-III-R was designed to be compatible with ICD-9-CM. Another factor was the argument by proponents of
the manual's revisions for the need to incorporate new scientific and clinical
findings from mental health. Because the DSM-III was such a major and extensive revision of the classification and diagnosis of mental disorders, proponents of the revisions argued that the ambiguities in DSM-III needed to be
cleared up as soon as possible for scientific and medical purposes.

Current treatment of mental illness as organic diseases of the brain (and
not problems in the psyche) as reflected in the DSM-III, DSM-III-R, and
DSM-IV played an important role in psychiatry's move back to claiming a
medical status. The resurgence of the medical model within psychiatry has
also been portrayed as a professional response to criticism from the labeling and antipsychiatry perspectives.

"ANTIPSYCHIATRY," LABELING, AND PSYCHIATRY'S RESPONSE

The success of post-World War II psychiatry's move away from the asylum and into the larger community and the expansion of treatments for a
range of behaviors considered "normal" were not without critics. There
were two intellectual and social movements in the 1960s and 1970s that
critically examined psychiatry: the antipsychiatry movement and the labeling perspective of mental illness.

The so-called "antipsychiatry" movement came out of psychiatry itself—as exemplified in the works of Thomas Szasz and R. D. Laing. According to this view, diagnoses are merely the way that the medical
profession deals with people who have "problems in living." Szasz argues
that the mind is not a bodily organ. Therefore, the term "mental illness" is
inappropriately affixed to misbehavior, not to a disease of the brain (Szasz
[1961] 1974). According to Szasz, mental illness is not a "bona fide" illness
because "[i]f mental illness is a metabolic or neurological disease, then it is
a disease of the body, not of the mind; and if mental illness is misbehavior
then it is behavior, not disease" ([1963] 1989:ix–x).

The labeling perspective on mental illness comes out of the symbolic interactionist school of sociology. Like "antipsychiatry," some psychiatrists consider it an "attack" on psychiatry and its classification of diagnoses (see Blashfield 1984). In the 1960s, sociologists Schatzman and Strauss argued for a clinical perspective that did not accept as "given" the legitimacy of psychiatric practice or mental illness. They note that "it would be much more fruitful for sociology if more research were done about psychiatry than in it or for it" (1966:4).

The labeling perspective focuses on the role of psychiatry (and other agents of "social control") in deciding and enforcing which behaviors are considered normal in conventional society. Sociologists and proponents of labeling theory ask the question: Who has the power to label people deviant?[3] Mental illness is considered a socially constructed *measure* of people's behaviors and not a true mirror of a reality that is happening within people's bodies or minds. How does some behavior get labeled as mental illness by doctors, lawyers, police officers, and the state? According to Scheff (1984): "[m]ental illness may be more usefully considered to be a social status than a disease, since the symptoms of mental illness are vaguely defined and widely distributed, and the definition of behavior as symptomatic of mental illness is usually dependent upon social rather than medical contingencies" (Scheff 1984:90).

By the end of the 1980s and during the time in which the LLPDD controversy occurred, three important sociological articles were published on the DSM-III and III-R and the psychiatric profession's turn to medically based psychiatric diagnosis. Loring and Powell's case study of psychiatrists and the DSM diagnoses they gave to patients found significant gender and racial variations (1988). In other words, men and women and blacks and whites were given different diagnoses by the psychiatrists, even though the "objective" case criteria were the same. The authors concluded that "even with carefully drawn standards, diagnosis will remain a subjective activity" and that "a false sense of confidence in objective measures can be dangerous when it ignores the possibility of bias (or misperception) and when it helps to maintain that bias through both treatment and statistical reports" (1988:19).

In a highly controversial article, Mirowsky and Ross took psychiatrists to task for using psychiatric diagnosis as "reified measurement."[4] They countered with the idea that "diagnosis as a form of measurement hinders understanding" of people's psychological problems (1989:12). According to Mirowsky and Ross, psychiatry in the 1980s began to promote diagnosis as *the* way to measure psychological problems. The DSM-III and DSM-III-R are examples of the APA's belief that "psychiatric entities exist" (1989:17). The authors point to the rise in biological psychiatry, and its desire to "look and sound like other medical specialties" as the primary reason for growing interest in creating and revising psychiatric diagnoses (1989:21). Other reasons include structural pressure from government agencies, insurance companies, and the pharmaceutical industry (Mirowsky and Ross 1989:22).

Another critic of psychiatric diagnosis is Phil Brown (1987, 1990). Based upon his systematic observation of a walk-in clinic, Brown observed that contrary to the popular image of the DSM-III as systematic and reliable, "[d]iagnostic work is full of conflict and contradiction" (1987:38). But it is the "chief language by which psychiatric and other medical reality is constructed" (1987:43). Using observational data, Brown shows how any psychiatric diagnosis is not just one phenomenon. A diagnosis has diverse functions and meanings for various groups such as insurance providers, government agencies, professional groups, and patients. Brown concludes that "it is precisely the inaccuracy of diagnosis, in its restricted DSM-III sense, throughout the mental health field that calls into question the validity of diagnosis, therefore producing and heightening diagnostic uncertainty, ambivalence, and conflict" (1987:49).

Brown's recent paper (1990) develops a more comprehensive sociological approach to the study of diagnosis in that it seeks to establish a research agenda for a future sociology of psychiatry. According to Brown, "the critique of diagnosis is the critique of psychiatry, because the diagnosis is the language of psychiatry, which by extension defines the practice of psychiatry" (1990:389 [143]). Brown emphasizes the need for sociologists to focus upon diagnosis because "[d]iagnosis locates the parameters of normality and abnormality, demarcates the professional and institutional boundaries of the mental health system, and authorizes psychiatry to label and deal with people on behalf of society at large (or, more appropriately, certain sectors of society)" (1990:289 [143]).

Brown also challenges the DSM-III-R: "[e]specially in the guise of DSM-III-R (American Psychiatric Association 1987), psychiatric diagnosis is the social representation of psychiatric knowledge, as well as the psychiatric profession's presentation of self" (1990:389 [143]). He suggests that the "remedicalization" of psychiatry by the proponents of biopsychiatry and the official diagnostic framework of the DSM-III and DSM-III-R are responsible for psychiatry's enlarged role in the social control and labeling of behavior.

As might be expected, psychiatrists have responded to the antipsychiatry and the labeling theory of mental disorders in a professionally adversarial manner. In addition to public relations campaigns to increase the visibility and status of the profession, the psychiatric profession responded to attacks by the antipsychiatry and labeling theory movement by once again specifically tying the profession with modern medicine.[5] I have shown in this last section that the development of the DSM-III and DSM-

III-R served as vehicles to reinforce psychiatry's ties to medicine by making mental disorders a subset of bodily disorders. As I explore in Chapter 9, DSM-IV continued along this path.

SUMMARY

Why do we need to be concerned about the psychiatric association and the development of the DSM? Tavris, psychologist and critic of the DSM, suggests that

> It is important to understand the claims, intentions, and methods of the DSM because the manual has had an extraordinary impact, both in the United States and worldwide. It has succeeded in standardizing the categories of who is, and who is not, mentally ill. Its categories and terminology have become the common language of most clinicians and researchers. Virtually all major textbooks in psychiatry and psychology base their discussions of mental disorders on the DSM. Insurance companies require clinicians to assign their patients the appropriate code number of the diagnosed disorder. Attorneys and judges often refer to the manual's list of mental disorders, even though the DSM warns that its categories 'many not be wholly relevant to legal judgements,' such as those of individual responsibility and competency. . . . The Manual generates a yearly revenue of over one million dollars for its publisher, the American Psychiatric Association. (Tavris 1992:178)

Interested professions such as psychiatry, psychology, and even sociology have long tried to stake claims for their unique perspectives on humans and the world (Freidson 1970a,b; Schacht and Nathan 1977; Brown 1987). PMS and the LLPDD controversy provide a site for exploring the questions of nature versus nurture and who should investigate and claim expertise in this area. I explore the claims between professions concerning LLPDD in greater detail in Chapter 4. Yet, claims to expertise and knowledge are also subject to historical and contemporary debate and changes within these professions. That is what is examined in this chapter. The history and the development of the APA tell us about how people with mental problems are perceived and treated in Western culture and, specifically, within North America. The development and recognition of LLPDD as a psychiatric disorder do not seem odd or out of place when connected to this history. The DSM and its revision process influenced the introduction of LLPDD. The introduction and acceptance of LLPDD are not out of line with the epistemological and professional changes that occurred in American psychiatry in the latter half of the twentieth century. As American psychiatry changed so did the emphasis on the classification of mental distress as a disease, a move away from social explanations for human behavior.

NOTES

1. Ironically, Grob points out that the initial impetus to classify psychiatric disorders came as a result of the rise of social sciences and the need to empirically document the number of people who had mental problems for the United States Census (1994).

2. In my interview with him, Spitzer also asserted that he does not like to label himself as a Neo-Kraepelinian.

3. Historians have been particularly important in documenting the politics of social control and the psychiatric profession. See works by David Rothman, *The Discovery of the Asylum: Social Order and Disorder in the New Republic* (1971), Andrew Scull, *Museums of Madness: The Social Organization of Insanity in Nineteenth-Century England* (1971), and Constance McGovern, *Masters of Madness: Social Origins of the American Psychiatric Profession* (1985). For a discussion of gendered social control, see Elizabeth Lunbeck, *The Psychiatric Persuasion: Knowledge, Gender, and Power in Modern America* (1994).

4. See the responses by psychiatrists and other sociologists to Mirowsky and Ross in the same volume of the journal.

5. The profession of psychiatry and membership in the APA remains strong. At the time of publication of the DSM-III-R in 1987, the APA membership totaled 32,000 (Encyclopedia of Associations 1987). In 1989 (the first year this information was published), the annual operating budget was listed at 20 million dollars. Today, the APA has a membership of approximately 39,000 members and an annual operating budget of 24 million dollars (Encyclopedia of Associations 1995).

3

The Narrative:
From PMS to PDD to LLPDD

Starting from the premise that neither scientific facts nor medical diagnoses are exempt from sociological analysis, LLPDD is the result of diverse social, economic and historical contexts and meanings. As indicated in Chapters 1 and 2, there were cultural and organizational forces that helped to shape the introduction of this new psychiatric diagnosis. In this chapter, I examine the people and events surrounding the American Psychiatric Association's decision to include a premenstrually related diagnosis in the DSM-III-R (American Psychiatric Association 1987). It is a narrative of how Premenstrual Dysphoric Disorder (PDD) came to be considered as part of the revision of DSM-III-R, how it quickly became controversial, and how debate was provisionally resolved by twice changing the name of the diagnosis and by locating it in an appendix. My narrative is based on extensive data collection from both public and private records, personal interviews, and published accounts of the controversy (explained further in the Introduction). It presents a stabilized, ex post facto description of what happened, who was involved, why there was an issue, where the events took place, and when they occurred.

THE NARRATIVE

In May 1983, the Board of Trustees of the American Psychiatric Association formally approved the creation of a Work Group to Revise DSM-III (hereafter referred to as "The Work Group") and appointed Dr. Robert Spitzer of the New York Psychiatric Institute as the Work Group chair.[1] Spitzer's appointment came following the recommendation of the Committee to Evaluate DSM-III to "fine tune" the DSM-III. Publication of the DSM-III-R was scheduled for mid-1985 (Spitzer and Williams 1987b:425).

The appointment of Robert Spitzer to chair the Work Group was somewhat predictable. He was no stranger to diagnostic revisions of the DSM and had been deeply involved in the DSM revision process and in the creation of contemporary psychiatric classifications and diagnoses (see Blashfield 1984). He played an important role in settling the 1973 controversy over deleting homosexuality from the DSM-II, and in adding ego-dystonic homosexuality in DSM-III (Bayer 1987; Kirk and Kutchins 1992). He also chaired the committee to revise DSM-II, which produced DSM-III.

The Work Group to Revise DSM-III met on May 3, 1983 in New York for an orientation and had its first full meeting on June 16, in Washington, D.C.[2] The group contained mental health professionals and scientists (mostly psychiatrists and a few psychologists). The APA's charge to the Work Group was to clarify ambiguities, resolve any inconsistencies, and incorporate factual changes and new cultural syndromes based upon scientific data that had accumulated since publication of the DSM-III in 1980.

By November 1984, Spitzer and the Work Group had drafted a working document that recommended the formation of needed scientific advisory committees and the proposed dates for their meetings.[3] Twenty-six specialized advisory committees were established to assist the Work Group in evaluating specific disorders. As the head of the Work Group, Spitzer chaired all 26 advisory committees. This document listed a new diagnosis, "Premenstrual Depressive Disorder," for possible inclusion in DSM-III-R.[4]

Spitzer appointed the "Premenstrual Advisory Committee" to help "work up" a premenstrual disorder category in DSM-III-R. When asked when the idea for a PMS diagnosis first came into being, Spitzer recalls:

I don't remember the date. I know how it happened. The way it happened was I would get invitations to conferences on PMS. And I, it just occurred to me at some point, 'Hey here's all this interest in this condition, that mental health professionals organize conferences on and although I don't know very much about the condition it seems as if the symptoms of the condition are primarily behavioral and mood changes. And if this really is a syndrome and affects women and it causes distress in some of them, how come this isn't being presented as a mental disorder?' Now that comes out of two interests: one, my job of trying to get into the classification all the disorders that people think are important or at least up for consideration. That's the part of the job that I saw that I had—which is, if there's been a description of some condition, there's been research on it and clinicians seem to think it's valuable in some context to diagnose it, then it would be up for consideration. The other interest that I've always had is what is a mental disorder. And I got that because I'm involved in the homosexuality thing. So having given a lot of thought to what is a mental disorder, in my own mind I had clearly decided that ideology was of no issue. So it was of no concern to me whether PMS had or did not have some kind of biological affinity. The issue for me just was, was it really an independent . . . did it have some validity as an independent behavioral syndrome. So, and that's how. So with that thought, I then touched base with people at NIMH . . . and we arranged that first meeting and that's how it started. (personal interview, May 23, 1991, New York City)

The APA and National Institute of Mental Health (NIMH) Center for the Study of Affective Disorders co-sponsored the June 1985 meeting of this committee. According to Spitzer, the members were selected in consultation with the staff of the Clinical Research Branch of NIMH.

In addition to Spitzer and Janet Williams (the text editor for DSM-III-R), 11 people were originally chosen to serve on the Premenstrual Advisory Committee. Sally Severino joined the Advisory Community after the June 1985 meeting.[5] All members of what became the LLPDD Advisory Committee were either research or clinical scientists with expertise in the area of premenstrual syndrome. They were

Judith Abplanalp, Ph.D.   Roger Haskett, M.D.
Susan Blumenthal, M.D.   Howard Osofsky, M.D., Ph.D.
Jean Endicott, Ph.D.   Barbara Parry, M.D.
Ira Glick, M.D.   Harrison Pope, M.D.
Jean Hamilton, M.D.   David Rubinow, M.D.
Wilma Harrison, M.D.   Sally Severino, M.D.

In the introduction to DSM-III-R, Spitzer and Williams explain that there were two main considerations in adding a new diagnostic category: Did the proposed category meet the requirements of the DSM-III definition of a mental disorder[6] and how compelling was the research or clinical need for the new category? The Advisory Committee's primary role was to advise the Work Group on whether a premenstrually related diagnosis met these requirements. If the committee recommended inclusion, a subcommittee would be chosen to work intensively on the diagnosis (personal interview, Robert Spitzer, May 23, 1991).

Initially, the committee postponed the decision on whether to include a PMS-related diagnosis in the DSM-III-R in favor of discussing the scientific criteria for such a diagnosis:

Recognizing that several members might have reservations about the merits of including a version of PMS in DSM-III-R, the issue of whether or not to recommend inclusion of the category in DSM-III-R was postponed until the committee had first drafted an initial set of criteria for cases of PMS in which mood disturbance was an essential feature. This draft definition would serve as the basis for the discussion about whether or not to include it in the manual. (Spitzer et al. 1989:893)

The name attached to the criteria was "Premenstrual Dysphoric Disorder" (PDD) instead of PMS to signify that psychological symptoms of the syndrome are unpleasant mood states or dysphoria (Spitzer et al. 1989).[7]

According to one anti-inclusion member of the Advisory Committee, this standard account by the Chair of the committee is not entirely accurate. Jean Hamilton believes that the "deck was stacked" from the start because a majority of those selected for the committee were already in favor of making PMS a psychiatric disorder (personal interview, June 4, 1990, Washington, D.C.). Hamilton's anti-inclusion beliefs served as the catalyst for fights over the diagnosis, because she arranged for a representative of the APA's Committee on Women to be present at the June 1985 meeting of the Premenstrual Advisory Committee.

Teresa Bernardez, a nonvoting representative and Chair of the APA Committee on Women, was "alerted" before the meeting by Jean Hamilton about the possibility of a PMS-related diagnosis (personal interview, April 20, 1990, East Lansing). Bernardez went to the meeting to present the Committee on Women's objections to including such a diagnosis. She offered two main critiques, which later became the core of the opposition stance throughout the controversy: first, the diagnosis would stigmatize all women; and second, there were insufficient scientific data to support inclusion (personal interview, April 20, 1990).

In spite of these initial objections, all but two members of the Advisory Committee voted for the inclusion of PDD in the DSM-III-R:[8] Hamilton voted against inclusion and research psychologist Judith Abplanalp abstained (Spitzer el al. 1989; Severino and Moline 1989). When pressed later for her position, Abplanalp went on the record as opposed to inclusion.[9]

BEGINNING THE CHALLENGE

Although their objections did not affect the Premenstrual Dysphoric Disorder Advisory Committee's vote, the Committee on Women continued to fight inclusion of PDD in DSM-III-R. Bernardez and Hamilton spent the months from June to September 1985 writing memos and letters, making radio and television appearances (e.g., National Public Radio segment on June 23, 1985), and attending meetings concerning PDD and two other controversial diagnoses proposed for inclusion in DSM-III-R: Paraphilic Rape Disorder and Masochistic Personality Disorder (Caplan [1991, 1995] and Caplan et al. [1992] discuss all three controversial diagnoses). The APA Committee on Women requested a formal liaison to the Work Group to be more fully informed about diagnoses pertaining to women.[10] Bernardez also requested participation rights for herself and other members of the

Committee on Women at the September Board of Trustee's (BOT) meeting to voice their objections to the diagnoses.

While the APA Committee on Women continued to challenge the process from within the APA, they also contacted other groups concerned with women's health and other related women's legal and social issues, hoping to get them involved in protesting the inclusion. Proponents of the diagnosis recall that it was during this time that "opponents of the category, representing many professional groups, mounted a vigorous campaign against its inclusion that included letters, petitions, and use of the mass media" (Severino and Moline 1989:22).

On September 16, the first of the groups outside the psychiatric association, the American Psychological Association Committee on Women, formally registered its opposition to the diagnosis. In a letter from the chair, Hortensia Amaro, the committee contended that "the diagnosis has ominous implications for perpetuating damaging stereotypes of women and for fostering an unnecessarily pathological view of women's experience."[11]

Another important group objecting to PDD (and the other controversial diagnoses) was the National Coalition for Women's Mental Health (NCWMH). Advised by Jean Hamilton, the NCWMH began to mobilize its efforts against the diagnoses by creating a "Task Force on Diagnosis."[12] Hamilton worked in conjunction with the APA Committee on Women, the NCWMH and later the newly formed Coalition Against Misdiagnosis (CAM) to publicize news about the possible inclusion of the three controversial diagnoses. Hamilton and her associates at the Institute for Research on Women's Health in Washington, D.C. compiled "briefing books" composed of women's expert analyses of each diagnoses.[13] "Action Alert" notices were sent to interested parties; petitions were started at women's health centers across the United States and Canada and the names and addresses of the leaders of the APA and Spitzer were publicized so letters of protest could be written.[14]

By early September 1985 it had become clear to Spitzer that opposition to PDD was serious and gaining ground. In a letter to the DSM-III-R Work Group, he wrote: "Several feminist groups, including the APA Committee on Women, have objected to our proposed inclusion of a new category of Premenstrual Dysphoric Disorder, recommended by an advisory group of researchers in this area. I will be meeting with the APA Committee on Women to see if we can handle some of their concerns about possible stigmatization of women by disclaimers in the text."[15]

The chance for Spitzer to meet with the Committee on Women came at the APA Board of Trustees' September Meeting a week after this letter was written. The topic of potential changes to DSM-III was last on the agenda.[16] At this meeting, the Committee on Women presented their objections to the inclusion of PDD as well as the two other controversial diagnoses. In a letter to the Work Group, Spitzer described the meeting:

> As they say in diplomacy, we had a 'frank exchange of views,' which means that we had some very serious differences. . . . Their main concern is with Premenstrual Dysphoric Disorder, which they feel will only stigmatize women and in no way encourage attention to women's special health needs. The fact that nine of the eleven experts on our Advisory Committee strongly supported the inclusion of this category in DSM-III-R does not impress them, and they have started to mobilize other groups (such as the American Psychological Association's Committee on Women) to start a campaign that would block the addition of this category.[17]

The Board of Trustees responded to Spitzer's acknowledgment of "the controversy that is now beginning with the Committee on Women" by appointing the Ad Hoc Committee to Review DSM-III-R of the Board of Trustees and Assembly of District Branches (hereafter Ad Hoc Committee). The Ad Hoc Committee was chaired by the APA's president-elect Robert Pasnau, and then later by Paul Fink. It was established to review the Work Group's progress and to pay attention to the proposed controversial revisions. The committee was composed of members of the Board of Trustees and the Assembly of District Branches.[18] The first meeting on the controversial diagnoses was scheduled for December 5 and 6, 1985.

Several events related to the controversy occurred during November 1985. At the November (15 through 17) meetings of the APA Assembly of District Branches representatives held a heated discussion on whether to even continue with revising DSM-III. The Assembly voted to recommend to the Board of Trustees that "APA put on hold target publication dates for a revision of DSM-III."[19] However, this recommendation was not supported by the Board of Trustees at their December meeting, and the revisions to DSM-III continued on schedule.

The second major event in November concerned a meeting of the Work Group with those opposed to inclusion of the diagnosis of Masochistic Personality Disorder.[20] Opposition forces included representatives from the Committee on Women, the American Psychological Association's Committee on Women, and other experts in the area of battered women and spouse abuse. The result of the meeting was the Work Group's decision to change the name of the diagnosis to Self-Defeating Personality Disorder and to add a companion diagnosis of Sadistic Personality Disorder, in spite of continued objections from the above groups (for differing accounts of this meeting see Brown 1985 and Goleman 1985).

Finally, in a letter dated November 27, 1985, the Association of Women Psychiatrists (AWP) registered their formal opposition to the inclusion of the controversial diagnoses. The AWP is not affiliated with the APA and is distinct from the APA's Committee on Women. In a one-page statement from their Executive Council, the AWP presented a summary of their objections to PDD.[21] These included premature classification, not enough research supporting the inclusion, the impeding of legitimate research on PMS if PDD is included, the coverage of the gynecological diagnosis of Premenstrual Tension Syndrome in the *International Classification of Diseases* (ICD), and the negative implications of using a psychiatric label to blame the victim.[22]

THE AD HOC COMMITTEE AND THE BOARD OF TRUSTEES

The first meeting of the Ad Hoc Committee took place on December 4 and 5—immediately before the December meeting of the Board of Trustees. The Ad Hoc Committee heard evidence from experts on both sides concerning the three controversial diagnoses. According to Bernardez, there was about an hour for the discussion (pros and cons) of the controversial diagnoses. The Ad Hoc Committee then adjourned to meet privately with the Work Group.[23] The following day the Ad Hoc Committee recommended to the Board of Trustees that Masochistic Personality Disorder (under the name Self-defeating Personality Disorder),[24] Sadistic Personality Disorder,[25] and Paraphilic Coercive Disorder (formerly Paraphilic Rapism) be included in the main text of the DSM-III-R. The committee recommended that Premenstrual Dysphoric Disorder be placed in an appendix and not the main text of DSM-III-R.[26] According to the account in *Psychiatric News*, "[c]iting the complex controversies surrounding the diagnosis, Pasnau's group had recommended including it in an appendix, if at all, and adding physical symptoms to the criteria" (January 3, 1986:24). The reasons for the addition of physical symptoms were based upon the observation that "Premenstrual Syndrome is included in ICD-9; and recommended that if it is included in any part of DSM-III-R, accompanying physical symptoms should be noted."[27]

On December 7, 1985 the Board of Trustees accepted the recommendations of the Ad Hoc Committee on all the diagnoses—except PDD. Citing the lack of time to review the issues involved, the Board decided against making a decision about the placement of PDD in either the main text or an appendix.[28]

TIME TO REGROUP

The goal of getting the DSM-III-R published was central to Spitzer. PDD and the other controversial diagnoses threatened its publication, as evidenced by the Assembly's recommendation to suspend publication due to the controversy. The Work Group's response to the Board of Trustees' decision was outlined in a letter to Bernardez dated 2 weeks after the Board of Trustees' meeting in December. Spitzer stated how he wanted public debate about the controversial diagnoses to proceed:

> I now believe that it would be a serious mistake for us to try to resolve the issue of these three controversial categories before there has been ample time for discussion and reflection. Since these three categories are in no way involved in the overall structure of the DSM-III-R, they could be eliminated shortly before the final document is approved. I therefore believe it will be useful for us to have discussion of these categories for a period of up to one year before a final decision will need to be made.[29]

As a result, Spitzer began to organize a symposium for a discussion of the controversial diagnoses at the May 1986 Annual Meetings of the APA, in preparation for the Board of Trustees' final decision about inclusion to be made at their June Meeting.[30]

The time from January 1986 to the Annual Meeting of the APA in May 1986 was apparently quiet. Beneath the surface was a full slate of events and efforts by both sides to mobilize resources and allies. The scientific press had been attracted to the controversy. For example, one hint of the simmering controversy is found in the January 24 "News and Comment" section in *Science* magazine, under the title: "Proposed New Psychiatric Diagnoses Raise Charges of Gender Bias" (Holden 1986). This article summarizes the events of the fall 1985 Ad Hoc Committee meeting and the positions held by the various "camps." It was an important marker because the controversy had now moved to a larger playing field, the press.

At the March Board of Trustees meeting, the issue of the placement of PDD was brought up by Pasnau who "reminded the Board that it deferred action to this meeting."[31] The Board voted to defer this matter until their June meting. It was also during the spring of 1986 that the Joint Research Council, the policy-making division of the APA, voted to recommend that the Board of Trustees drop PDD from DSM-III-R.[32]

The Annual Meeting of the APA was held in May 1986 in Washington, D.C. This is where the controversy heated up and entered the *public* realm as a result of publicity generated by protests held inside and outside of the convention center. Although descriptions of the Annual Meeting varied somewhat depending upon which source is read, they all focused upon the controversy over the diagnoses. By various accounts, the meeting was (1) business as usual—nothing really happened except a few "ubiquitous protestors picketed outside largely unnoticed" (*Psychiatric News*, June 6, 1986:18), (2) taken over by angry feminists protesting against the inclusion of a few diagnoses deemed damaging to women (popular press, newspapers), or (3) mostly concerned with the various scientific and medical issues and symposium related to the controversial diagnoses in DSM-III-R (see Staver 1986a).

What *did* happen at this meeting? On May 13, protestors from the Feminist Therapy Institute (FTI), the Coalition Against Misdiagnosis (CAM), and individual members of the Association of Women Psychiatrists (AWP) picketed the outside of the convention center and spoke out against the diagnoses. Inside the convention, Spitzer and the APA were holding their own press conference on the controversial diagnoses. According to CAM member Lenore Walker:

> [t]heir response to our protest was to invite us to hold a joint press conference inside the Convention Center. So, after our Speak-Out, we all dramatically filed in there to hear Bob Spitzer tell us that the Work Group is thinking of dropping Paraphilic Coercive Disorder from consideration but is still committed to keeping the others. . . . Sally Severino, M.D. defended the use of the PMS category so women could find out whether or not they had such cyclical mood swings! Psychologist Paula Caplan and psychiatrists Marjorie Braude, Jean Baker Miller and Alexandra Symonds (Chair of the Awp), articulately defended the feminist position. They were clear to point out to the press that every major mental health group and women's group have all taken the same position against the APA's[33] process and diagnostic decisions.[34]

Later that day, the symposium that Spitzer had earlier proposed to Bernardez in December was in fact held. "Symposium 43: Controversies in the Revision of the DSM-III" played to a packed audience. Under the title "Premenstrual Dysphoric Disorder in DSM-III-R Will Stigmatize Women," Jean Hamilton and Sheryl Alagna [Gallant] spoke for the "Affirmative" and Barbara Parry and Sally Severino for the "Negative" sides of the question. This debate, along with the press conference, was fully covered by the media and resulted in numerous articles and commentaries about the controversy with titles such as "Is PMS Mental Illness? Debate Grows" (Carey 1986), and "Cursed and Pre-Cursed" (nationally syndicated column by Ellen Goodman, May 24, 1986). It also received much attention in newsletters by the Feminist Therapy Institute, Association of Women Psychiatrists, and the Coalition Against Misdiagnosis.

Another important event took place at this meeting. Robert Pasnau, who had been serving as the chair of the Ad Hoc Committee, took office as the President of the APA. In his Presidential Address, Pasnau referred to the controversy over PDD and the other disputed diagnoses. He declared:

> [t]here is probably nothing that has a greater impact on our public image than the validity and reliability of psychiatric diagnoses. For instance, the inclusion of premenstrual dysphoric disorder in DSM-III-R not only affects our members and their women patients but has an influence on the public trust

in psychiatry as well. We must be mindful of this interaction between science, economics, and public image. (as quoted in *Psychiatric News* June 6, 1986:5)

Anti-inclusion protestors took this statement as a good sign that their objections were finally being heard.

THE FINAL MONTHS OF THE CONTROVERSY

After the APA Annual Meeting, the action shifted to the Board of Trustees. At their June 28, 1986 meeting, the Board heard presentations by the APA Committee on Women (Bernardez and Nada Stotland, the new chair of the committee) and members of the Work Group and the Ad Hoc Committee. They then voted to put the PMS-related diagnosis Self Defeating Personality Disorder and Sadistic Personality Disorder in the appendix of DSM-III-R. The name of the PMS diagnosis was officially changed from Premenstrual Dysphoric Disorder (PDD) to Periluteal Phase Dysphoric Disorder (PLPDD). According to Spitzer et al., this was done to recognize that there are "a small number of cases that occur in women who are not menstruating" (1989:893). Further, Spitzer stated that the changed name "avoids somewhat the stigmatization of the 'curse'" (as quoted in Keyser 1986).

In the official announcement of the vote in an APA press release, President Pasnau is quoted as saying that the Board was "not yet convinced that the scientific evidence, while impressive, is sufficiently strong to warrant inclusion in the text of the manual at this time." However, Periluteal Phase Dysphoric Disorder and the two other controversial diagnoses "are of sufficient clinical importance to justify publishing them in the appendix to the manual for research and educational purposes."[35]

The press portrayed the Board's decision as "surprising" and "shocking" because it went against the advice of its own Advisory Committees, the Work Group, and the Ad Hoc Committee. This was true of Self Defeating Personality Disorder and Sadistic Personality Disorder, but not of what was then renamed Periluteal Phase Dysphoric Disorder. The Advisory Committees and the Work Group pushed for inclusion of all the diagnoses in the main text (interview, Robert Spitzer, May 23, 1991). However, the Ad Hoc Committee had recommended an appendix for what was then Premenstrual Dysphoric Disorder, and including the other two diagnoses in the main text of DSM-III-R in December 1985. The Board of Trustees' decision to place all three of the controversial diagnoses in an appendix also went against the Ad Hoc Committee's overall recommendations in December 1985.

The APA's Committee on Women remained opposed to inclusion of all three of the diagnoses even in the appendix. In terms of PLPDD, they argued specifically in their official statement that "scientific evidence was still lacking for a premenstrual syndrome diagnosis, considering its potential for stigmatizing women by linking a psychiatric disorder with the menstrual cycle" (as quoted in *Psychiatric News*, July 18, 1986:7). The inclusion of the other two controversial diagnoses in the appendix was considered a small victory because the decision went against the Ad Hoc Committee's earlier recommendation of inclusion in the main text.

For the Work Group, the Board's decision was considered to be a defeat (personal interview, Robert Spitzer, May 23, 1991). Spitzer's stated public reaction was that "if the Board opposed the work group's recommendations, it would be the first time the Board, a political body, had told a technical group what to include" (*Psychiatric News*, July 18, 1986:7). Although the Board's decision appeared to be final, it was not yet binding and more decisions and issues about the nature of the appendix, whether code numbers would be given and if a cautionary statement was needed, were still up for negotiation.

By August 1986, the second draft of DSM-III-R was available and circulated among interested psychiatrists and nonpsychiatrists. Periluteal Phase Dysphoric Disorder appeared in two different places: in the main text with a reference to the appendix ["See Appendix A: New Controversial Categories in DSM-III-R"] and also in Appendix A. The main text reference to PLPDD infuriated members of the Committee on Women. They began the fight to strike any reference to PLPDD (and the other controversial diagnoses) in the main text.

There was also considerable disagreement over whether a diagnostic code number would be assigned to the categories in the appendix.[36] Why was the code number such an important issue? A code number in the DSM makes the diagnosis even more "real." The disorder could be referred to, given to women, and possibly used for insurance, legal, and diagnostic purposes. The second draft of DSM-III-R listed PLPDD with the code number 307.90 [Periluteal Phase Dysphoric Disorder].[37] The Committee on Women fought the assignment of any code other than a "V" code [for "conditions not attributable to a mental disorder that are a focus of attention or treatment" (American Psychiatric Association 1987:9]. The Committee on Women charged that any code other than a "V" code would constitute PLPDD as a regular diagnosis. They argued that it was the first time any diagnosis in an appendix had a numerical code and that it would be the same as having the diagnosis in the main text of the DSM-III-R.

The Committee on Women had a new chair, Nada Stotland. Stotland was prepared for the possibility of having the diagnosis carry a regular code number, but continued to press for the total elimination of the diagnosis.[38] Spitzer and the Work Group, on the other side, continued to push for the assignment of a regular code, but seemed willing to compromise to avoid the possibility of "total appendectomy" of the diagnosis.[39] According to Spitzer, having the diagnosis in the appendix with a code number was a compromise that the Work Group was willing to live with:

> If it's in the appendix people can use it. Also by giving it a code number, yeah, I mean once we realized it had to be in the appendix we did the best to elevate it within the appendix. So like by giving it a code number that was one way of saying, 'you can still use this category if you want.' There was no statement that you couldn't use it. (personal interview, Robert Spitzer, May 23, 1991)

In November 1986, there was one last major skirmish over the inclusion of the PMS-related diagnosis in DSM-III-R. At the November meeting of the Assembly of District Branches, Area III (for Washington, D.C.), representatives presented an action paper calling for the deletion of the appendix and the three controversial diagnoses from the DSM-III-R. This move to delete the appendix was defeated, and the Assembly of District Branches voted to approve the final draft of DSM-III-R.[40] The Assembly did, however, vote to bar any reference to the controversial categories in the main text.[41]

The Board of Trustees accepted and approved the final draft of DSM-III-R in December 1986. The Board agreed to place the three controversial diagnoses in the appendix under the heading "proposed diagnostic categories needing further study." It also voted to strike any reference to these disorders from the main text. In the battle over the code number, however, the Work Group won. The code number assigned to Periluteal Phase Dysphoric Disorder was 307.90: Other and Unspecified Special Symptoms or Syndromes, Not Elsewhere Classified.[42]

The DSM-III-R appeared in May 1987, 2 years after its projected completion date. By this time, the diagnosis of PLPDD had been transformed by this time into Late Luteal Phase Dysphoric Disorder (LLPDD). According to Spitzer et al., the name was changed to recognize that "strictly speaking, the symptoms were not 'around' ("peri') the luteal phase but actually occurred during the late luteal phase" (Spitzer et al. 1989). The name changes were the result of discussion with gynecologists and PMS researchers. As Spitzer recalls:

> I think what happened was we felt Premenstrual Dysphoric Disorder sounded too much like PMS. So then we thought, 'okay, let's do more scientific—Periluteal. And, then I think after the Board actually used that term, somebody pointed out that Periluteal is not as accurate as Late Luteal, so then we changed it. (Personal interview, May 23, New York City)

It is interesting to note that in the alphabetic and numerical listings in the DSM-III-R (Appendices G and H), the code number LLPDD was 307.90 as defined by the Board of Trustees. However, in the text of the diagnostic criteria for LLPDD Appendix A, researchers and clinicians are told to assign code number 300.90 (Unspecified Mental Disorder, Late Luteal Phase Dysphoric Disorder). In addition and contrary to the directions of the Board of Trustees, there is a reference to LLPDD in the main text. Under the final section of the main text titled "Additional Codes," the following explanation is given for code 300.90 (Unspecified Mental Disorder, Nonpsychotic):

> In some cases with more information the diagnosis can be changed to a specific disorder. This category can also be used for specific mental disorders that are not included in the DSM-III-R classification, for example, Late Luteal Phase Dysphoric Disorder. (American Psychiatric Association 1987: 363)

The phrase "specific mental disorders" suggests that even though it is not listed in the official DSM-III-R classification, LLPDD was real enough and could be recorded using the 300.90 code number for insurance and diagnostic purposes.

CONCLUSIONS

The narrative account of the controversy over inclusion of a PMS-related diagnosis reads as a story of one artifact (LLPDD) and one controversy that took place primarily over a 3-year time period from 1985 to 1987. Lost in this particular form of presentation is the multiplicity of divergent interpretations of the events as they happened, by different participants. The rest of this book is designed to recover these divergent interpretations and accounts in the later chapters and to analyze them with the tools of constructivist sociology of science, feminist critiques of science and medicine, and social science models of the professions.

NOTES

1. Memo dated April 20, 1983 from Drs. Brodie and Tarjan to Dr. Spitzer, in American Psychiatric Association Archives, Washington, D.C.
2. Memo from Spitzer, May 16, 1983 in American Psychiatric Association Archives, Washington, D.C.
3. Document titled "Meetings Sponsored by the Work Group to Revise DSM-III in American Psychiatric Association Archives, Washington, D.C.
4. Document titled "The Process of the Revision of DSM-III" dated November 29, 1984 in American Psychiatric Association Archives, Washington, D.C.

5.   Dr. Severino was asked to be on the committee due to her clinical expertise and recent scientific studies done with women with PMS. She went on to became an important person in the debate and controversy through her public appearances, letters to editors, and participation in the debate at the APA Annual Meeting in May 1986.

6.   According to the DSM-III-R, a mental disorder is "a discrete entity with sharp boundaries (discontinuity) between it and other mental disorders, or between it and no mental disorder" (American Psychiatric Association, 1987:xxii).

7.   By naming the disorder PDD instead of PMS, the committee was also providing differentiation of the psychological states of the disorder from biological states necessary in order to be included in DSM-III-R, a distinction that proves to be an important issue as the controversy unfolded.

8.   The vote was eleven to two. This does not add up to the members of the Advisory Committee due to the later addition of Dr. Sally Severino after the June 5, 1985 meeting. Dr. Severino was an active supporter of the diagnosis.

9.   Because Abplanalp was an active PMS researcher at the time of the vote, Hamilton believed that Abplanalp's vote against the inclusion of the diagnosis could have proved harmful, i.e., in getting her research funded by the National Institute of Mental Health (whose scientists were among the leading proponents for the inclusion of LLPDD) (interview with Hamilton, June 4, 1990).

10.   Letter from Dr. Teresa Bernardez to Dr. Robert Spitzer, dated July 2, 1985, American Psychiatric Association Archives, Washington, D.C.

11.   Letter to Dr. Robert Spitzer from Hortensia Amaro, Chair of the Committee on Women in Psychology, dated September 16, 1985 in The American Psychiatric Association Archives, Washington, D.C.

12.   Letter from Jean Hamilton to Robert Spitzer, July 17, 1985. Personal records of Dr. Jean Hamilton, Institute for Research on Women's Health, Washington, D.C.

13.   Copies of these booklets and related documents are found in Dr. Jean Hamilton's personal records, Institute for Research on Women's Health, Washington, D.C.

14.   This process started in the Fall of 1985 and the results were successful if judged only by the volume of petitions, letters of protest, and telegrams sent by individuals and professional groups to the APA leaders, Dr. Spitzer and Dr. Bernardez. They have been deposited in the American Psychiatric Association Archives, Washington, D.C.

15.   Letter from Dr. Robert Spitzer to members of the Work Group whom he called "Revisionists" dated September 10, 1985, American Psychiatric Association Archives, Washington, D.C.

16.   Document titled "Agenda of BOT's September Meeting," American Psychiatric Association Archives, Washington, D.C.

17.   Letter from Dr. Robert Spitzer to "Revisionists" dated September 25, 1985, American Psychiatric Association Archives, Washington, D.C.

18.   According to Barton (a former president of the APA), there are four major bases of power in the American Psychiatric Association that need to be considered in any of its decisions: The President and the Board of Trustees, which are "the ultimate authority" in the APA; the Assembly of District Branches, which "derives its power through member-elected representatives from the District Branches"; the

Medical Director of the APA, who "inevitably filled the role as Association leader"; and the Joint Reference Committee "with the authority to accept, reformulate, or reject policy recommendations emerging from groups of experts" (Barton 1987:284, 290).

19.　For a full account of this meeting and action, see *Psychiatric News*, December 6, 1985:1.

20.　This was important because the campaign against DSM-III-R launched by the Committee on Women tied all the diagnoses that affected women together.

21.　Position statement of AWP sent to Dr. Robert Spitzer, dated November 27, 1985, American Psychiatric Association Archives, Washington, D.C.

22.　The issue of compatibility with the International Classification of Diseases is explored in depth in Chapter 5.

23.　Undated report to the Committee on Women by Dr. Teresa Bernardez, personal records of Dr. Jean Hamilton, Institute for Research on Women's Health, Washington, D.C.

24.　The change of name was made at the meeting about Masochistic Personality Disorder held by the Work Group to Revise DSM-III in November 1985 prior to the Ad Hoc Committee meeting. The meeting was attended by the Work Group and opposition forces from the Committees on Women from both the psychiatric and psychological associations and other experts in this area.

25.　At the November 1985 meeting held by the Work Group to Revise DSM-III, this diagnosis was suggested as a complementary diagnosis to Masochistic Personality Disorder.

26.　Memo written by Dr Roger Peele, Vice-Chair of Ad Hoc Committee, dated December 6, 1985, American Psychiatric Association Archives, Washington, D.C.

27.　From a document titled "Unofficial Highlights of a Meeting, December 6–7, 1985," American Psychiatric Association Archives, Washington, D.C.

28.　Letter from Peele to Dr. Jean Hamilton and others, dated December 18, 1985. Personal records of Dr. Jean Hamilton, Institute for Research on Women's Health, Washington, D.C.

29.　Letter from Dr. Robert Spitzer to Dr. Teresa Bernardez, dated December, 1985. Personal records of Dr. Jean Hamilton, Institute for Research on Women's Health, Washington, D.C.

30.　Letter from Dr. Robert Spitzer to Dr. Teresa Bernardez, December 1985. Personal records of Dr. Jean Hamilton, Institute for Research on Women's Health, Washington, D.C.

31.　Page 17 of document titled "Report to Staff Cabinet on March'86 BOT," American Psychiatric Association Archives, Washington, D.C.

32.　There are references to this decision found in various sources, such as an undated Joint Research Council memo, American Psychiatric Association Archives, Washington, D.C and the CAM newsletter, June, 1986.

33.　Psychologists use the acronym "ApA" and "Awp" to denote the psychiatric association as opposed to their own organization the American Psychological Association, also the "APA".

34.　Coalition Against Misdiagnosis Memo titled "Update and Report on Washington DC" dated May 20, 1986, personal records, Dr. Jean Hamilton, Institute for Research on Women's Health, Washington, D.C.

35.   APA press release dated June 28, 1986. American Psychiatric Association Archives, Washington, D.C. (see also Lander 1988:15).

36.   Memo for the APA Committee on Women, personal records, Dr. Jean Hamilton, Institute for Research on Women's Health, Washington, D.C.

37.   "Second Draft: DSM-III-R in Development" dated August 1, 1986, Work Group to Revise DSM-III, American Psychiatric Association Archives, Washington, D.C.

38.   Letter from Dr. Nada Stotland to Dr. Jean Hamilton dated November 6, 1986. Personal records of Dr. Jean Hamilton, Institute for Research on Women's Health, Washington, D.C.

39.   Letter from Robert Spitzer to "Revisionists" [Work Group Members] dated September 1986. American Psychiatric Association Archives, Washington, D.C.

40.   As reported in *Psychiatric News*, December 5, 1986.

41.   Letter to Board of Trustees from Robert Spitzer, dated November 28, 1986, American Psychiatric Association Archives, Washington, D.C.

42.   As reported in *Psychiatric News*, January 2, 1987.

II

The Three Domains of Conflict

4

Accounting for the Controversy

The narrative account of LLPDD and the DSM-III-R in Chapter 3 provides the necessary background information about a recent scientific and political controversy. The story is based upon research and the collection of empirical data, but otherwise includes no explicit sociological analysis. It can be read as "factual" without assigning privilege to the analyst—aside from having in her possession more obscure or nonpublic data.[1] I begin the sociological analysis of the LLPDD controversy by examining and criticizing three readily available public accounts that other people have used to explain the events. I then suggest a theoretical alternative for examining this and other controversies by paying attention to the issue of the "ownership" of social problems and employing a social worlds perspective.

MULTIPLE ACCOUNTS OF LLPDD

Figure 4.1 presents the final criteria for LLPDD. Here it is seen as a finished product; in this form, LLPDD is owned and copyrighted by the American Psychiatric Association. When examined as a finished product and taken out of the context of the people, events, and actions that compose the controversy, LLPDD is just another psychiatric diagnosis with set criteria, a ready-made fact. In this form, the diagnosis does not appear so controversial, nor does it seem sociologically interesting. At the time of its construction, about 5% of women were stated to be severely affected by premenstrual symptoms and thought to qualify for the diagnosis of LLPDD (Blumenthal and Nadelson 1988; Spitzer et al. 1989; Gold and Severino 1994). LLPDD *existed*, psychiatrists *diagnosed* it, and women *had* it or they *did not*.

The first step toward a sociological analysis of this controversy is to examine how LLPDD was represented in various settings (e.g., public versus private, medical journals versus the popular press) and by different people concerned about LLPDD (e.g., reporters, psychiatrists, scientists,

Figure 4.1. Late Luteal Phase Dysphoric Disorder as found in Appendix A of DSM-III-R.

A. In most menstrual cycles during the past year, symptoms in B occurred during the last week of the luteal phase and remitted within a few days after onset of the follicular phase. In menstruating females, these phases correspond to the week before, and a few days after, the onset of menses. (In nonmenstruating females who have had a hysterectomy, the timing of luteal and follicular phases may require measurement of circulating reproductive hormones.)

B. At least five of the following symptoms have been present for most of the time during each symptomatic late luteal phase, at least one of the symptoms being either (1), (2), (3), or (4):

 (1) marked affective lability, e.g., feeling suddenly sad, tearful, irritable, or angry
 (2) persistent and marked anger or irritability
 (3) marked anxiety, tension, feelings of being "keyed up," or "on edge"
 (4) markedly depressed mood, feelings of hopelessness, or self-deprecating thoughts
 (5) decreased interest in usual activities, e.g., work, friends, hobbies
 (6) easy fatigability or marked lack of energy
 (7) subjective sense of difficulty in concentrating
 (8) marked change in appetite, overeating, or specific food cravings
 (9) hypersomnia or insomnia
 (10) other physical symptoms, such as breast tenderness or swelling, headaches, joint or muscle pain, a sensation of "bloating," weight gain

C. The disturbance seriously interferes with work or with usual social activities or relationships with others.

D. The disturbance is not merely an exacerbation of the symptoms of another disorder, such as Major Depression, Panic Disorder, Dysthymia, or a Pesonality Disorder (although it may be superimposed on any of these disorders).

E. Criteria A, B, C, and D are confirmed by prospective daily self-ratings during at least two symptomatic cycles. (The diagnosis may be made provisionally prior to this confimation.)

Note: For coding purposes, Record: 300.90 Unspecified Mental Disorder (Late Luteal Phase Dysphoric Disorder). Copyright © 1987 The American Psychiatric Association, used with permission.

women with PMS). What are these accounts, who is making them, and how and why are they different?

There were three readily available and reductionistic interpretations of the LLPDD controversy: (1) the *economic account*, in which LLPDD is the result of the APA's economic interests in the DSM; (2) the *political account*, in which LLPDD is the result of simple political interests and power; and (3) the *rational account*, in which LLPDD is seen as the product of rational bureaucratic and scientific procedures.

AN ECONOMIC ACCOUNT

The first account that explains why LLPDD was proposed for inclusion in the DSM-III-R was economic. Charges were leveled (both within and outside the APA) that the decision to revise DSM-III was based solely on financial considerations—that the APA would gain monetarily from the requirement that members of the mental health community purchase the new DSM-III-R (Fisher 1986). For example, when DSM-III-R was published in 1987, 120,000 copies were sold within a 6-month time period at a publishers's price of approximately $36. By its fifth printing in September 1988, the APA Press had printed 360,000 copies of the manual (book jacket, DSM-III-R). By the end of 1992, the DSM-III and the DSM-III-R had sold at least 1,600,000 copies with translations into 11 languages (McCarthy and Gerring 1994). Critics also argued that the APA was devising new disorders to justify the revision process and to expand its client base (at the expense of other medical and mental health professionals).

This economic issue was brought up in debate among APA members and the press accounts of DSM-III-R revisions numerous times. For example, at the November 1985 meeting of the APA Assembly, a few members of the Assembly asked if the revision was being 'rushed' into print because of the sizable revenues its sales would bring (as discussed in *Psychiatric News*, December 6, 1985:6). In the course of the LLPDD controversy, this charge was brought up and discussed at length within the APA and in the popular press. According to a spokesperson for the APA during the debate (President-elect Robert Pasnau), the decision to revise DSM was not based on financial considerations—but if the revision process were stopped, as opponents tried to achieve, the financial repercussions would have been severe.

In the minutes of the Joint Reference Committee (JRC), Pasnau stated that the "[c]laims that the APA is revising DSM-III for income purposes are false although, if DSM-III is halted at this stage, there will be serious financial implications"[2] (undated minutes of the JRC, Spring, 1986). This sentiment was echoed in the Annual Report of the Medical Director of the APA, Melvin Sabshin. Sabshin stated in defense of the DSM-III-R:

> One specific concern I have had about some of the debates on DSM-III-R relates to assertions by some members that the primary motive for DSM-III-R has been economic gain for APA to the detriment of many of the members. . . . Nevertheless, planning for DSM-III-R preceded these budgetary projections, and all involved perceived an updating of DSM-III as a useful scientific and professional project. Indeed, I have frequently spoken and written about DSM-III as a reflection of psychiatry's clearer boundaries and scientific status. (Sabshin 1986:1342)

In spite of serious public allegations about the economic reasons for revising the DSM and a vote by the Assembly of District Branches to reevaluate the revision process, the work on DSM-III-R and LLPDD continued.

In terms of LLPDD, many of the letters of protest written to Spitzer and APA leaders (explored in depth in Chapter 6) made the connection between possible economic benefits accruing to psychiatrists and the proposed diagnosis. For example, one woman wrote: "The recent attention to PMS seems like just another quick illness to make money off of, after it has been ignored for so many years" (letter of protest, dated June 3, 1986). Another woman answered the question "Why is this being done?" with the answer "I suspect an economic reason—not a medical one. No doubt someone stands to make more dollars from insurance if the name is changed [from PMS to LLPDD]" (letter of protest, dated July 21, 1986). Finally, one woman ended her letter by stating: "I realize that the new labeling would cultivate for psychiatrists a new area for getting insurance reimbursements given only for diseases sanctioned by the Diagnostic and Statistical Manual. I hope that this does not bias any decisions" (letter of protest, dated July 12, 1986).

The economic accounts placed the explanation for the revision of the DSM-III and for the proposal to include LLPDD in the DSM-III-R in very simple terms. The APA was economically motivated to publish the DSM-III-R and justified the new edition by proposing new diagnoses. Psychiatrists would also benefit economically through insurance reimbursements by claiming PMS (as manifested in LLPDD) as a psychiatric disorder.

THE POLITICAL ACCOUNT

As shown in Figure 4.2, a very simple *political account* is also available to explain the controversy: Premenstrual Dysphoric Disorder, which was

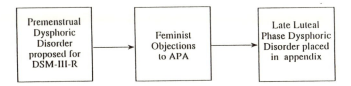

Figure 4.2.   The standard political account.

the original name for the diagnosis, met with the political objections of "feminists," which resulted in changing the name of the disorder to Late Luteal Phase Dysphoric Disorder and placing it in an appendix.

This account provided a short and simple explanation for the controversy. Who opposed it: feminists. Why did they oppose it: they were feminists—which implies that "feminists" opposed it only for political reasons and not for scientific reasons. Explanation for the controversy is narrowed to a simplistic political accounting of the events. The scientific issues about the definition of PMS, and professional opposition from the American Psychological Association and all of the major mental health groups, are all ignored.

I provide four examples of this accounting: First, then Vice President of the APA, Dr. Paul Fink, described and summarized the objections of feminists in an introduction to the written proceedings of a major PMS conference:

> Much of the controversy that ensued had little to do with the diagnostic category or the condition itself. Rather, it concerned feelings voiced by feminist groups that the new diagnostic category would be misleading, that it would inappropriately label women as mentally ill, and that it would be affixed not only to the dysphoric disorder, but everything else that happens psychiatrically to women.[3]

From another source, a respected handbook on psychiatry, the essentially political nature of the controversy is expanded upon as the ubiquitous "feminists" are equated with "some women":

> A revised edition of the DSM-III was published in 1987 (DSM-III-R). . . . Some new categories were added. One was Late Luteal Phase Dysphoric Disorder, hormonalese for premenstrual syndrome. Some women object to premenstrual syndrome being called a psychiatric disorder. Changing the name was intended to appease them but didn't. They picketed APA headquarters and held long sessions with lawyers. The term got in anyway, but in a Needing Further Study section.[4]

Examples of this political account were also prevalent in the popular press. An example ran in a Washington, D.C. newspaper, under the headline, "APA Cuts Manual to Please Feminists":

> Feminist opposition to listing several controversial new diagnostic categories in a national manual of psychiatry caused one of them to be dropped and the others to be relegated to the less official back of the book. . . . Critics of a diagnosis for premenstrual syndrome argued it would stigmatize women and resurrect old perceptions that women are unstable during their monthly 'curse.'[5]

In this account, not only did feminists object to the inclusion, but they were directly responsible for and thus "caused" the diagnosis to be placed in an appendix.

I also found a political account of the controversy and settlement in the official newsletter of the American Psychiatric Association, *The Psychiatric Times*. The following anonymous impressions of psychiatrists were recorded in a report of the June 1986 Board of Trustees action to place LLPDD in an appendix:

> A nationally prominent psychiatrist, insisting on anonymity, said, 'The Board of Trustees seems to have an unerring instinct for public relations fiascoes and self-destructive ambivalent obsessions. This mess doesn't help psychiatry at all.'[6]

So, in the hands of some participants (like Drs. Fink, Goodwin, and Gaze) and journalists (like Lucy Keyser and the anonymous psychiatrist), there was nothing complicated about LLPDD: psychiatrists proposed a move that ran against the perceived interests of women; feminists and women's groups protested; a *political* compromise was reached, and into the appendix it went.

This public representation of objections to the inclusion of LLPDD as primarily "feminist" was important in the debate for the following reasons. The labeling of the opposition as "feminist" was crucial in portraying the issue as political and not one of inconclusive science. This portrayal undercut the arguments of some psychiatrists, scientists, and psychologists by calling them feminists, thus taking away the cultural and professional authority of their arguments (which were ironically based upon the scientific merit of the proposed diagnosis). In the quotation from *The Psychiatric Times*, this is clearly represented in the charge that the Board of Trustees "capitulated to feminist political pressure." This simplistic explanation obfuscates or ignores arguments by opponents of the diagnosis about the *scientific* validity of construct (see Chapters 6 and 7 for further discussion of this representation).

THE RATIONAL ACCOUNT

Another explanation of the controversy—one used by proinclusion psychiatrists—situates it narrowly within the organizational decision-making machinery of the APA, within the DSM revision process, and within advances in scientific research. The representation of the LLPDD controversy offered by these participants in the controversy is one that is a rational, scientific, and bureaucratic fact.

Figure 4.3 represents the rational accounting of the controversy within the context of a timeline of the events as they happened blow-by-blow within the APA. In the same way that the standard political account reduces LLPDD to an "inevitable" and "uncomplicated" political struggle between feminists and the APA, this chronological picture makes it seem as though the eventual outcome unfolded rationally and bureaucratically, as various bodies within the APA successively collected new information and made sequenced decisions according to a rational bureaucratic procedure. Interestingly, most of the examples of the rational account that I could find were made *after* the controversy had taken place and settled. The rational account constitutes an ex post facto legitimizing explanation and served to stabilize the outcome. The outcome, i.e., to place LLPDD in an appendix, is here seen as the most reasonable, judicious, and even inevitable decision. In addition, the controversy is portrayed as giving PMS some well-defined criteria in LLPDD, and thus a scientific "linear" improvement over previously established National Institute of Mental Health guidelines for its definition.

One document that provides this explanation of the controversy is the DSM-III-R. The following statement about LLPDD and the "Appendix for Proposed Diagnostic Categories Needing Further Study" was included in the introduction of the DSM-III-R, and written by Robert Spitzer and Janet Williams:

> This controversy was resolved by the inclusion of these three categories in Appendix A: Proposed Diagnostic Categories Needing Further Study (see p. 367). They are not listed in the Classification of Mental Disorders, but are included in the manual to facilitate further systematic clinical study and research. (American Psychiatric Association 1987:xxv–xxvi)

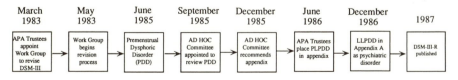

March 1983	May 1983	June 1985	September 1985	December 1985	June 1986	December 1986	1987
APA Trustees appoint Work Group to revise DSM-III	Work Group begins revision process	Premenstrual Dysphoric Disorder (PDD)	AD HOC Committee appointed to review PDD	AD HOC Committee recommends appendix	APA Trustees place PLPDD in appendix	LLPDD in Appendix A as psychiatric disorder	DSM-III-R published

Figure 4.3.   The rational account.

Another attempt to explain the controversy in rational bureaucratic terms is found in the introduction to a special edition of *The Journal of Clinical Psychiatry* on LLPDD and Premenstrual Syndrome. The authors provided the following explanation:

> The controversy and debate were resolved by including the disorder in the Appendix section of the DSM-III-R. This approach permits the diagnostic criteria to be used to achieve consistency in definition of the syndrome for both clinical and research purposes until more research evidence is accumulated that either validates or negates the utility of this diagnostic construct. (Blumenthal and Nadelson 1988:471)

This explanation is interesting since the authors were both active participants in the debate and controversy. Susan Blumenthal was a proinclusion scientist from NIMH and an LLPDD Advisory Committee Member; Carol Nadelson was president of the APA during the early months of the controversy.

In another version of this explanation of PMS and LLPDD, authors Michael Gitlin and Robert Pasnau discuss the methodological problems in PMS research:

> The proposed DSM-III-R criteria for PMS, defined as late luteal phase dysphoric disorder, attempt to circumvent many of these methodological difficulties [related to PMS research]. Late luteal phase dysphoric disorder is classified as a proposed category needing further study. (Gitlin and Pasnau 1989:1416)

This accounting is important in light of the position within the APA of one of the co-authors. Robert Pasnau served as Chair of the Ad Hoc Committee, President-elect, and President of the APA during the years of the controversy. The scientific potential of LLPDD as a psychiatric disorder is emphasized by pointing out that inclusion of LLPDD in the appendix has paid off in scientific advance. Gitlin and Pasnau conclude that

> Although validity cannot be assumed from reliability, the adoption of operational criteria, such as recently proposed for late luteal phase dysphoric disorder in DSM-III-R, helps to clarify some basic nosological questions in these disorders. (1989:1420)

The inclusion of LLPDD in Appendix A is portrayed as not only politically beneficial but also as scientifically and clinically beneficial for the advancement of knowledge. For example, in my interviews with two leading proponents for inclusion of the diagnosis in the main text (Severino and

Spitzer), both psychiatrists pointed out that although they were initially opposed to the idea of an appendix, it was ultimately useful in yielding studies that show the scientific validity and clinical applicability of the diagnosis. According to Spitzer:

> Oh now there are a lot of very good studies which give a prevalence of 3 or 4 percent, which is nice, you know, from our viewpoint of what's what. I think it's a prevalence that it's high enough that you can say 'hey, this is something significant. It's not one in ten thousand. It's not some exotic condition.' On the other hand, it's not so common that you would say, we'll just diagnose it. So yeah, those studies are very supportive. I mean, the whole situation nowadays is very different than it was three years ago. (personal interview, May 23, 1991, New York City)

The emphasis in the rational account on research criteria and clinical implications of placing LLPDD in an appendix is further exemplified in a recently published PMS book. Allen Frances, the chair of the committee to create DSM-IV, wrote the following in the introduction to a book on PMS co-authored by Sally Severino:

> The decision for DSM-III-R was to include a category with the cumbersome name Late Luteal Phase Dysphoric Disorder within the appendix of the manual, but not to give it official status in the nomenclature. This was meant to promote research on the disorder, while minimizing possible misuse of the diagnosis.[7]

If the political accounting puts all of the explanatory weight on the colliding interests of feminists and the APA, this rational accounting appears to leave out interests altogether. The decision to include LLPDD in an appendix of DSM-III-R results from a fair and judicious settlement in the delegation of bureaucratic and scientific responsibility for PMS—all according to rational, logical procedures.

As suggested by the already existing multiple accounts or explanations of the controversy, no single accounting can effectively explain how and why LLPDD was controversial and ended up in the appendix of DSM-III-R. The accumulation and translation of scientific evidence into mental health policy are not just economically motivated, a political outcome, or a "rational and logical" process. LLPDD took on many different meanings during the controversy. But how can we examine the multiple meanings attached to LLPDD by the various people who had different and shifting interests during the controversy? The concept central to this book is the "ownership" of social problems and the perspective is the "social worlds" perspective in the sociology of science.

OWNERSHIP, DOMAINS AND SOCIAL WORLDS

Figure 4.4 summarizes graphically three domains in which the battle over the ownership of PMS and LLPDD was fought. The shaded area in the center points to the issue of PMS—which is what the three domains have in common. As suggested in the introduction, actors struggled for what Joseph Gusfield has called "the ownership" of a social problem, that is, who has to right to define, control, and benefit from a particular definition of the problem. PMS and LLPDD were not just issues for the two opposing groups, but for a constellation of often overlapping actors and social groups. All were trying to claim ownership of PMS and its psychiatric manifestation in LLPDD.

The ownership claims come out of "social worlds"—when collective actors share similar outlooks, concerns, and commitments (Strauss 1978; Becker 1982). I use the term "domain" to locate and distinguish the multiple social worlds involved in the contested arena of LLPDD and PMS. This term allows for spatial understanding of the location of the actors and distinguishes the multiple meanings of the controversial fact or artifact. Conflict and controversy arise when people from different social worlds hold different perspectives about the way something should be defined, pursued, or created (Fujimura 1988; Clarke 1990a). This is what happened in the LLPDD controversy. But the question arises: if different actors have different meanings of the artifact under construction or contestation, how can you distinguish and locate the social worlds in relationship to one another?

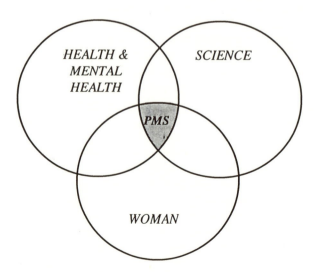

Figure 4.4.   The three domains of PMS/LLPDD.

Domains are constructed by the actors in the controversy and the sociological analyst (myself in this case) who is making the connections between what the actors say, do, or are implicated in the struggle. Thus, a domain is simultaneously (1) a place of social interaction where people and their shared interests in the fact or object interact; and (2) a theoretical and analytic construct that is fashioned by the analyst of the controversy and guided by work and theory in sociology. The actors and groups involved in the LLPDD controversy "are not only those individually and collectively 'present,' articulate, and committed to action in that arena but also those implicated by actions in that arena. That is, the actions taken in that arena will be consequential for them, regardless of their current presence, organization, or action" (Clarke and Montini 1993:45). The inclusion of sociological analysts as actors into the social worlds is also necessary to give the reader a more comprehensive picture of the way in which objects and truth are debated and resolved. The constructed nature of LLPDD is further shaped by locating it within situated sociological knowledges. Each of these situated knowledges turns LLPDD into three objects during the controversy over its inclusion in the DSM-III-R.

THE THREE DOMAINS OF PMS

Identifying and constructing the public (newspaper, official explanations in journals and books, and press releases) versus the private accounts (personal interviews and documents) of the controversy was an important step in my analysis of the LLPDD controversy. One of the most important hidden pieces of information about LLPDD is that the first and primary opposition to the diagnosis came not from outside "feminist groups" (as the press accounts portrayed) but rather from the APA's own Committee on Women. Most of these women would describe themselves as feminists; they are also eminent psychiatrists and scientists. This suggests that they would have a variety of sometimes conflicting interests in PMS. Intensive focus upon the actions and strategies of the Committee on Women (i.e., the Committee on Women served as an analytical "wedge") enabled me to "fashion" or "make" the three distinct but overlapping domains of the LLPDD controversy. By focusing initially on this committee and talking to the two psychiatrists (Hamilton and Bernardez) who spearheaded opposition forces, the shape of my analysis of the controversy began to change.

First, the Committee on Women chose to go outside the APA and enlist other health, mental health, and legal professionals in creating an alliance to fight the inclusion of the diagnosis. I have called this the *health and mental health* domain. In doing this, the Committee linked LLPDD to larger professional concerns in the definition and treatment of mental illness. They actively solicited support from organizations such as the American Psychological Association, the National Association of Social Workers, and the American Orthopsychiatric Association. Through strategies chosen by the APA's Committee on Women, LLPDD became the occasion for contests of professional dominance, raising questions about the hierarchy of authority in the health and mental health fields. As situated in sociological works on the professions and especially psychiatry, LLPDD is an artifact in which gynecologists, psychiatrists, psychologists, psychiatric nurses, and social workers were all struggling with one another to gain control of the health and mental health fields. I contend that LLPDD was at the center of shifting and ambiguous boundaries of contested professional terrain.

The Committee on Women also linked themselves to a variety of feminist and women's groups, for whom the diagnosis was not a "contest among professionals" but a struggle between experts and laity for control over women's bodies and minds: a struggle over the definition of a normal and healthy woman. This *woman*[8] domain included expert and professional women who made claims to speak on behalf of all women as well as individual women with PMS who claimed their own authority to speak for themselves. The crucially important APA Committee on Women took LLPDD into this domain as they pursued certain strategies to advance their initial interest in getting this "antiwoman" diagnosis completely removed from DSM-III-R. When situated in feminist theories and critiques of science, gender studies, and historical and anthropological studies of women and menstruation, LLPDD was a gendered artifact related to issues of stigmatization and control of women's bodies. It was the object in which the definition and control of what constitutes a normal and healthy woman were at stake. Feminist health, mental health, and political groups/individuals pitted themselves in a gendered struggle against the effect of labeling all menstruating women as potentially "crazy."

Finally, the Committee on Women also chose to ground their opposition to the inclusion of a PMS-related diagnosis on the argument that there were insufficient scientific data to warrant such a move. This strategy moved LLPDD into yet a third domain: science. Here, LLPDD was neither a contest among professions nor a struggle between women and experts, but rather an example of "nature" (the reality of PMS and LLPDD) that was still being negotiated. PMS and LLPDD became part of a larger struggle for control over the construction of scientific truth in the midst of a public controversy. In establishing LLPDD as a scientific fact and artifact, I situate the controversy in studies in the sociology, history, and philosophy of science and technology. LLPDD represents scientists constructing the reality of the natural world in the battle to define and control the scientific "truth" about PMS and LLPDD.

SUMMARY

A more traditional form of sociological analysis would look like the diagram in Figure 4.5: From the suggested diagnosis of PDD, three domains of conflict opened up and the result was LLPDD. But Star and Griesemer describe a situation in which "boundary objects" have "different meanings in different social worlds but their structure is common enough to more than one world to make them recognizable, a means of translation" (1989:393). As suggested in Figure 4.6, LLPDD was more than one artifact during the debate and controversy. The multiple constructions of LLPDD by the actors in the different domains of the controversy, by sociological literatures and by the analyst, make PMS as manifested in LLPDD three different phenomena. The analysis of domains shows that although the result of the controversy was "one" stabilized artifact in the DSM-III-R, there were three domains of conflict that initially produced three different LLPDDs. During the controversy, LLPDD was not one stable artifact but three distinctively different phenomena.

The distinctively different faces of LLPDD in the domains are presented and explained in more detail in this section of the book. Is LLPDD a simple case of constructed knowledge based only upon "interests" of certain powerful groups or a true representation of real, severe emotional symptoms of PMS? Examination of the data in three different domains allows the analyst and the reader to recognize that LLPDD is not just about interests, not just about power, and not just about whether it is a true reflection of the natural world. It is all of these. LLPDD has multiple realities. The decision to place LLPDD in an appendix served to stabilize the artifact and the controversy—both the DSM-III-R and Late Luteal Phase Dysphoric Disorder have been in the public domain since 1987.

Not to be lost in this kind of analysis are the broader sociological issues and methodological implications of this study. This study focuses upon the *ownership* of social problems and how this is tied to issues of power and control. LLPDD was deemed an important artifact by different social actors and groups who engaged in struggle with each other over the right to define and control PMS. As explored in the next three chapters of this book,

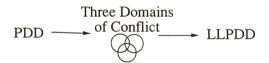

Figure 4.5. Traditional sociological conceptualization of LLPDD. In this type of analysis, LLPDD is the same object, which is the result of three domains of conflict.

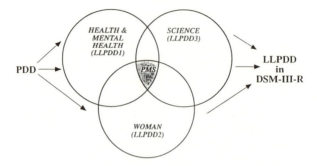

Figure 4.6.   Domain analysis of LLPDD controversy.

each party that claimed control over LLPDD used a distinctive power base (professional knowledge and expertise, personal experience, political perspective, and scientific expertise) to justify its authority to define the phenomenon.

The domain analysis offered here invites attention to significant and enduring sociological questions about the controversy and construction of scientific and medical artifacts: "Who is making these claims and why?" "On what grounds does a certain claim to truth exist?" and "How is this truth determined and settled?" The settlement of controversy certainly reflects the ability of some actors and groups to determine what becomes the accepted view of reality. It also reflects the social, political, and organizational processes through which this occurs. That these same processes can occur in *different* domains of interaction representing different artifacts and outcomes is a measure of the strength of this antireductionistic position.

NOTES

1.   This stabilized account is also a constructed version of what happened based upon different claims and sources of data. It is "factual" in the sense that it has been based upon and made by human activity (see Latour 1987).

2.   Joint Reference Committee Meetings, Spring 1986. American Psychiatric Association Archives, Washington, D.C.

3.   Forward to *Premenstrual Syndrome: Ethical and Legal Implications in a Biomedical Perspective*, Benson Ginsburg and Bonnie Carter (eds). 1986. New York: Plenum Press.

4.   Preface to Donald Goodwin and Samuel Guze, *Psychiatric Diagnosis*, fourth edition. 1989. New York: Oxford University Press.

5.   Keyser, July 4, 1986:80 in *The Washington Times*.

6.   August 1986 edition of *The Psychiatric Times*.

7.   Dr. Allen Francis in the forward to Sally Severino and Margaret Moline, *Premenstrual Syndrome: A Clinician's Guide*. 1989. New York: The Guilford Press.

8.   In spite of many comments or suggestions to use "women" or "women's" domain, I have stuck (however stubbornly) to using the term "woman." It is the vision and body of "everywoman" that is being debated in PMS. I have also been influenced by the monolithic "woman" that Emily Martin writes about in *The Woman in the Body* (1987) and that Carol Tavris speaks of in *The Mismeasure of Woman* (1992).

5

Inter- and Intraprofessional Boundary Disputes: The Health and Mental Health Domain

> Diagnosis is often the location in the psychiatric world where both lay and professional critics fight over the roles and functions of diagnoses. These struggles are ample proof that scientific discoveries are not the result of an ongoing 'march of science' as much as of political battles. (Brown 1990:403)

As the above quotation suggests, decisions about medical diagnoses often become battlegrounds for professional dominance and control among health and mental health occupations. In the "health and mental health domain," LLPDD is located at the center of shifting and ambiguous boundaries of this contested professional terrain. Professional boundary issues were established early in the controversy, when the APA Committee on Women actively solicited and received support from mental health groups inside and outside the American Psychiatric Association. The conflict over LLPDD focused the attention of participants and the public on issues of professional boundaries surrounding the *right* to define and treat PMS.

Sociologically, contests for professional dominance raise issues inherent in the division of labor among the health and mental health fields. Which profession has control over others in a given jurisdiction? How are the different levels of expertise and control divided up among health professionals of equal status? How are challenges to professional control made and settled? These sociological questions are answered in a number of ways in the health and mental health domain. The boundaries of the domain are first established by reviewing sociological theories of the professions, especially those developed in medical sociology. These are helpful in constituting LLPDD as an artifact of professional dominance. This domain of analysis is also constructed by examining public and private debates among health and mental health professions during the LLPDD controversy. This chapter explores why and how the APA responded to four challenges to defend their professional boundaries.

SOCIOLOGICAL THEORIES OF THE PROFESSIONS

What does the literature in the sociology of professions offer an analyst studying the LLPDD controversy? How does it constitute LLPDD as an artifact of professional dominance? Definitional standards of what and who constituted a "real" profession were matters of frequent discussion in early functionalist studies of professions (Carr-Saunders and Wilson 1933; Parsons 1939, 1958; Cogan 1953, 1955). There was general agreement that modern physicians constituted the apex by which all other professions would be judged. In the early 1960s and into the 1970s, debate turned to "professionalization" as a process that characterizes some—but not all—occupations. The focus shifted from definitions of what constitutes a profession to theories of how and why professions develop (Wilensky 1961; Bucher and Strauss 1961).

A more critical stance toward the professions and their role in society also characterized this time period. In 1970, Eliot Friedson changed the professions literature with two influential books, *Professional Dominance* (1970a) and *The Profession of Medicine* (1970b). He suggested that the study of professions (in particular, the modern medical profession) should focus on how some occupations assume a dominant position in the division of labor. For example, he indicates that in the division of labor in the medical care system, there are numerous conflicts among professionals in the struggle for dominance of the field (e.g, between physicians and nurses, or pharmacists and physicians).

Friedson extended the sociological assumption that medicine was a kind of exemplar among professions. In its connection to science and technology, physicians have surpassed other professions in prestige and in their dominance over other health care workers. The profession of medicine has come to be the "prototype" on which other occupations seeking privilege and power model their professionalizing quest. According to Friedson, the "better we understand medicine, then the better we will be able to understand the problems that may be posed by the professionalization of the key service workers of the welfare state" (1970b:xviii). Light recently summarized professional dominance theories of Friedson as the prevailing view of the professions in sociology. The model sees professions, especially medicine, "as an elite set of occupations which have somehow obtained state powers to monopolize their domain of work, train their own members, dominate the boards of certification and licensure that approve new members and related institutions (like hospitals), monitor their quality of their professional work, and run most of the institutions where their work takes place" (Light 1988:204).

The 1970s and 1980s marked the rise of critical, political economy studies of professions. The "monopoly" school of thought traced the links between professions and capitalism, imperialism, and other organizing features of the market. Whereas Friedson focused on monopolization and dominance within and among professional providers, the monopoly school showed that this happened within the capitalist economic system. Professions were portrayed as corporate groups engaged in mobility projects aimed at their control of labor and services (Larson 1977; Berlant 1974; Brown 1979). These works are critical of how modern professions have achieved the monopolization of their labor markets in modern capitalism, and how this is linked to the spread of imperialism and capitalism throughout the world.

Abbott's *The System of Professions: An Essay on the Division of Expert Labor* (1988) shows how professions "exist in an interrelated system." By focusing upon the *work* of a profession instead of its occupational organization, and by looking at the control and content of professional tasks, Abbott concludes that "[c]hanges in professions can therefore best be analyzed by specifying forces that affect the content and control of work and by investigating the disturbances in that content and control propagate throughout the system of professions and jurisdictions" (Abbott 1988:112). The public arena is one site in which interprofessional competition occurs, and in which claims to knowledge and expertise are fought out (1988:58).

FRAMING LLPDD AS A PROFESSIONAL DISPUTE

LLPDD and its controversy (from 1985 to 1987) is a site where professionals in the health and mental health fields made diverse claims about the definition of PMS and about its treatment. Hierarchies in the division of labor of both health and mental health occupations were salient for the outcome of the LLPDD controversy. Bucher and Strauss's (1961) emphasis on emergent groups *within* a profession (which change and influence that professional group) is highlighted by the role of the APA Committee on Women in the controversy. Abbott usefully points out the need for historical analyses and for studies of competition among rival professionals (1988). Abbott's model—which centers on disputes among professions over the jurisdictional control of work tasks—has much theoretical vitality for the analysis of the LLPDD controversy. He focuses precisely upon the *control* of knowledge and on how professions compete and battle for that control. Abbott's analysis is strengthened by including economic, social, and historical factors that play an important role in definitional boundary-setting: "[p]rofessionalization occurs, to be sure, but in a context that helps determine its course. A comprehensive theory of professional life must deal with these complex facts of jurisdictional competition and interprofessional relations" (1988:23).

Throughout the making of LLPDD, there were many disputes over responsibility and control in the "professional projects" of psychiatry and other health and mental health fields. I have drawn upon the definition of "project" by Larson (1977). The word "does not mean that the goals and strategies pursued by a given group are entirely clear or deliberate for all the members, not even for the most determined and articulate among them. Applied to the historical results of a given course of action, the term 'project' emphasizes the coherence and consistence that can be discovered ex post facto in a variety of apparently unconnected acts" (1977:6).

My focus on disputes among professionals is also influenced by Gieryn and his studies of science as a profession (1983, 1994). Gieryn asks: how can one know what science is? His answer is to focus sociological research on the occasions when the boundaries are negotiated and provisionally stabilized. Gieryn and his associates studied contests in which resources such as money, power, and professional control hang in the balance of such boundary-work [see Gieryn et al. (1985) for a study of two historically significant creation-science trials, Gieryn and Figert (1986) for a study of what happens when scientists cheat, and Gieryn and Figert (1990) for an analysis of the space shuttle Challenger accident investigation].

THE HEALTH AND MENTAL HEALTH DOMAIN ANALYSIS

As the review of the literature on the professions suggests, a sociological analysis in the Health and Mental Health Domain makes it possible (1) to show how LLPDD became an arena or site in which issues of professional dominance and jurisdictional expertise were contested among various health and mental health professionals; (2) to identify and describe groups and their interests involved in the conflict; and (3) to analyze how these groups interacted with each other and negotiated a settlement (albeit temporary) about PMS as manifested in LLPDD.

Who is to treat PMS and with what services/prescriptions? One of the more consistent charges leveled against the psychiatric association in the LLPDD debate was that psychiatrists were trying to recruit more patients from an otherwise shrinking pool and to make them eligible for insurance reimbursement for treatment of this "disorder." This charge was consistently denied by APA officials, but it points to the highly contentious nature of the professional debate over who should identify and treat PMS. LLPDD became a site in which health and mental health professionals debated and fought over the ownership of PMS. LLPDD created four major divisions: between psychiatrists and gynecologists, among different schools of psychiatric thought, in the hierarchy of the mental health professionals (i.e., psychiatrists, psychologists, social workers, and psychiatric nurses to name a few), and finally between mental health professionals and nonprofessionals such as nutritionists and drug companies claiming their own definitions and treatment capabilities. In each of the professional disputes in this domain, the boundaries of psychiatry were actively being challenged. How and why psychiatry as a profession responded to these challenges in the LLPDD controversy forms the basis for the analysis in this domain.

WITHIN THE MEDICAL PROFESSION

When Robert Frank in 1931 introduced his research on "premenstrual tension," he suggested that neurologists were the appropriate medical professionals to deal with the "large group of women who are handicapped by premenstrual disturbances of manifold nature" (1931:1053). He concluded that "careful study of the changes occurring in the autonomic nervous system, particularly such reactions as lend themselves to accurate analysis, be undertaken by *neurologists* at that time of the cycle at which symptoms of tension are most manifest" (Frank 1931:1057 [emphasis added]). Debate over inclusion of LLPDD followed a similar demarcation: both gynecologists and psychiatrists claimed that they were better suited to diagnose and treat women with severe premenstrual disturbances.

This conflict between medical specialties is best explained by going into an in-depth analysis of the conflict over whether what became LLPDD would carry a diagnostic code number in the DSM-III-R. As explained in Chapter 3, there was significant discussion about whether LLPDD would carry a code number, a V code, or no code at all. Obscured in this larger debate with the Committee on Women is the conflict and settlement between gynecologists and psychiatrists. When Premenstrual Dysphoric Disorder was first proposed as an addition to DSM-III-R, it carried with it the code number 625.40. This number was given to maintain compatibility with the list of diseases and mental disorders located in the World Health Organization's *International Classification on Diseases* (ICD-9-CM), which contains the category of "Premenstrual Tension Syndromes."

Premenstrual Tension Syndromes is listed under "Other Disorders of Female Genital Tract" in the ICD-9-CM chapter on "Diseases of the Genitourinary System." According to the ICD-9-CM, Premenstrual Tension Syndrome is "A group of physical and psychological symptoms which in varying combinations characteristically recur in women in the second, luteal phase of the menstrual cycle and subside during the first 11–12 days of the cycle. The commonest symptoms include tension, irritability, depression, painful breasts, fluid retention and backache. The relationship of mental ill-health and hormonal disturbance to this syndrome remains unclear" (W.H.O. 1989:33).[1]

The use of code numbers, and their compatibility with other diagnostic classification systems, became a major source of contention between gynecologists and psychiatrists during the LLPDD debate. The initial use of the code number for Premenstrual Tension Syndrome (625.40) to label Premenstrual Dysphoric Disorder caused a furor, because gynecologists claimed that psychiatrists were overstepping their professional boundaries. Psychiatrists' creation of a diagnosis with a gynecological code number led to a controversy over the right to define and treat PMS among members of the medical profession. In successive reformulations of LLPDD, the disorder was changed from a gynecologic to psychiatric code number to maintain the division of labor in the health care delivery system among medical specialties. Since both gynecologists and psychiatrists are medical doctors, the treatment and diagnosis of PMS as a psychiatric or gynecological disorder were significant issues. Given the "biological" realignment of psychiatry (to become closer to the medical profession), this dispute was an important boundary defining issue (see Chapter 2 for further explanation about this trend).

Gynecologists claimed that they were better suited not only to diagnose but to treat PMS because it was a physiological or biological disorder. The boundary dispute resulted in letters from gynecologists to the APA, protesting inclusion of a PMS-related diagnosis in DSM-III-R. One physician from Los Angeles wrote the following to the APA:

"How stupid can you get?! There is no wonder at all that the label, head shrinker (Shrink), is used. There is no significant justification (theoretical or practical) for any effort to classify the condition as a mental or emotional disorder." (dated June 26, 1986)[2]

From another gynecologist in Portland, Oregon:

The PMS issue strikes me as an obvious mistake. In my practice as a gynecologist I see many women who are quite obviously changed each month by their cyclic hormones.... The fact that we do not understand all the biochemical forces underlying these symptoms does not mean they don't exist, or that they s[h]ould be assigned to the Central Nervous System—your area. As long as gynecologists take care of endocrinologic problems of women, this is our province, not yours. (letter dated July 19, 1986)[3]

Physicians, and their professional associations, were wary that labeling PMS a "mental" disorder might preempt further biological research on a condition that was not obviously a psychiatric condition. A gynecologist who works with women with PMS wrote:

> Do we really want to label as psychopathology the expression of anger during the premenstrual phase? In addition, it is not always so clear-cut that the premenstrual emotional symptoms reflect a pathological state. There are some patients in whom the premenstrually expressed feelings may represent a greater state of health and insight than those expressed—or repressed—in the nonpremenstrual state. We are just at the beginning of understanding the interrelationship between a women's menstrual cycle and her emotional state. While I am sympathetic to those who would like to have a recognized psychiatric disorder to treat, this move is extremely premature in the case of PMS. (letter dated March 26, 1986)[4]

The argument that the diagnosis was based upon inadequate research, and that it resulted in stigmatization, was a popular one among nonpsychiatric physicians. Although not directly challenging the professional authority of psychiatrists to medically treat women, the gynecologists' arguments suggested a privileged position—as that specialty assumed the task of speaking for their women patients and for all women. From another doctor in Los Angeles:

> PMS should remain a gynecological diagnosis. There have been distressingly inadequate research studies exploring this entity. To add to the burden of these women who are afflicted with this problem, the additional burden of thinking of themselves (and having society and their therapists think of them) as disordered because they have mood changes in accord with hormonal changes does not seem helpful. There is not even any clear scientific evidence that a cause and effect relationship exists. (letter dated June 12, 1986)[5]

From the Greater Atlanta Physicians Association came the suggestion that even physicians have not reached consensus about the diagnosis:

> We believe that such a diagnosis is potentially discriminatory. In addition, there is no consensus in the psychiatric community that PMS is a mental illness. We oppose the inclusion of a PMS classification in the DSM III coding structure and hope you will reconsider this action. (letter dated April 14, 1986)[6]

This uneasiness over the lack of consensus was further evidenced by some psychiatrists who wished that the subject would remain in the gynecologists' realm of treatments and disorders:

> It is not a psychiatric disorder. The research literature on menstrual-related-cycle mood or behavior changes show inconsistent and contradictory find-

ings. In my personal observation I found that all male psychiatrists with expertise in the field found the diagnosis useful, while most of the women psychiatrists did not. (letter dated November 20, 1985)[7]

Another letter of protest was written by a psychiatrist in California, who declared that

Premenstrual Disorder is a gynecologic, not psychiatric, diagnosis. There are no useful studies documenting the diagnostic validity or implementation of this formulation. (letter dated June 5, 1986)[8]

A humorous but telling comment on Premenstrual Dysphoric Disorder came from a psychiatrist in Florida. He succinctly wrote:

Premenstrual Dysphoric Disorder, omit. Let the gynecologists worry over this bag of worms. The description is too involved and if you have them doing self-ratings you'll just make them [women] more neurotic. (letter dated November 27, 1985)[9]

Because of letters like these, the Work Group and other psychiatrists supporting inclusion of the diagnosis were forced to contend with the matter of intramedicine professional boundaries. Robert Spitzer, the Head of the Work Group to revise DSM-III, stated, in response to criticism that PMS is already a gynecological disorder, that "Gynecologists are totally irrelevant. This is purely a mental disorder. It is not a physical or neurological disease" (as quoted in Mickelsen, June 4, 1986).

Members of the Work Group and Advisory Committee repeatedly emphasized that LLPDD was consistent with the definition of mental disorders in DSM-III and DSM-III-R and as such is the province of psychiatrists (Robert Spitzer, personal interview, May 23, 1991; Sally Severino, personal interview, May 24, 1991). The DSM-III-R definition of a mental disorder is "a clinically significant behavioral or psychological syndrome or pattern that occurs in a person and that is associated with present distress (a painful symptom) or disability (impairment in one or more important areas of functioning) or with a significantly increased risk of suffering death, pain, disability, or an important loss of freedom" (American Psychiatric Association 1987:xxii).

Spitzer and other psychiatrists favoring inclusion also pointed out that the diagnosis of LLPDD unambiguously differentiates women with gynecological problems from those with severe psychological problems. According to Spitzer, "the diagnosis is justified in view of the fact that the majority of women who complain to their doctors are more distressed about the psychological than the physical symptoms" (as stated in Holden 1986:327). As LLPDD was defined by psychiatrists from the Work Group, not all women diagnosed as having PMS would qualify for the psychiatric diagnosis. The definition of LLPDD was restricted to "a subgroup of women with PMS whose symptoms are primarily affective (depression, mood swings, anger, anxiety) but restricted to the late luteal phase of the menstrual cycle. Symptoms must be so severe that they seriously impair the woman's functioning" (Severino and Moline 1989:9). According to their arguments, the skills and expertise of psychiatrists were required to differentiate PMS from LLPDD (as well as any other mental disorders). This is why, according to Severino, "[t]o me, this says that you need a mental health professional to make that differential diagnosis" (as quoted in Staver 1986a:26).

Another argument by proinclusion psychiatrists deflected the issue away from gender bias to a more immediate bias against psychiatry. They charged that the boundary uproar was largely due to a negative image of psychiatry and the possibly stigmatizing effect of labeling a psychiatric disorder (Severino, personal interview May 24, 1990). David Rubinow of the LLPDD Advisory Committee and a PMS researcher at NIMH stated that "[i]n this particular case, the controversy is largely reflective of the bias that exists in society not against women but against psychiatry and psychiatric disorders" (as quoted in Rovner 1987:8). Stemming from the antipsychiatry movement in the 1960s, bias against the psychiatric profession was seen as an important element in the debate, especially by the psychiatrists and scientists who supported the inclusion of LLPDD. As Spitzer stated: "There were some who were upset with it [LLPDD] but they would be as upset with almost any psychiatric diagnosis. They just don't like psychiatric diagnoses" (personal interview, May 23, 1991).

The diagnostic conflict between the two medical specialties was negotiated and eventually settled in the following manner. In the course of the controversy, the code number changed from 625.40 for Premenstrual Dysphoric Disorder to 307.90 for Periluteal Phase Dysphoric Disorder (in the second published draft of the DSM-III), and then to 300.90 for Late Luteal Phase Dysphoric Disorder (in the final published version of the DSM-III-R). In other words, the APA Board of Trustees changed the status of LLPDD as a diagnosis from a gynecologic to a psychiatric disorder by virtue of changing the code number of the diagnosis [from a gynecological code (625.40) to a psychiatric code (307.90) Late Luteal Phase Dysphoric Disorder and (300.90) Unspecified Mental Disorder]. In an explanation for the coding changes, Spitzer made the following comments:

> Look, there are a lot of different arguments made against the category. One argument is you already have that in gynecology so there's no. . . . you don't need this disorder. Psychiatrists, you know, if he [sic] wants to, he can always

use, he can diagnose it if he wants. So the argument against that is to say 'but this is not the same condition and it's not a gynecological disorder'. So, if you're going to argue that it's not a gynecological disorder, that it's a mental disorder then it's nonconsistent to give it a gynecological number. That's all. (personal interview with Robert Spitzer, May 23, 1991)

During the controversy, changes in the code number and the name of the disorder were linked as highlighted in the correspondence of Roger Peele, M.D., who served on the Work Group, was the Vice-Chairman of the Ad Hoc Committee, and was also Chair-Elect of the Assembly of District Branches during most of the controversy. In a letter to Spitzer immediately after the December 1985 Ad Hoc Committee meeting, Peele wrote of his discomfort in using the term "premenstrual" to describe the newly created disorder. He suggested using the words "cyclic" or "periodic" because, in his opinion, the word premenstrual suggests that a woman's uterus may be the cause of the disorder instead of the brain (letter from Peele, dated December 13, 1985).[10] In further correspondence with Spitzer, Peele suggested other possible names, and hints that gynecologists might even be jealous of the specificity claimed for "periluteal phase dysphoric disorder" (letter to Robert Spitzer, June 3, 1986).[11]

Peele's influence in getting the code number changed is evidenced in a letter from him to Jean Hamilton in which he states that he was able to convince Spitzer to change the code number from a gynecological disorder to a mental health disorder to avoid having psychiatrists making gynecological diagnoses (dated January 13, 1986).[12] This claim is confirmed in a letter from Peele to Stephen Sharfstein, M.D., at the APA.[13]

In his annual report to the APA as the Chair-Elect of the Assembly of District Branches, Peele publicly defended the action of renumbering the diagnosis as a psychiatric disorder rather than putting psychiatrists in the position of making a gynecological diagnosis. He explained that

> While my suggestion to change the code of premenstrual dysphoric disorder from a gynecological to a psychiatric one has been accepted, I am still opposed to premenstrual dysphoric disorder being a regular part of American psychiatric diagnosing. After physicians mistreated women for centuries with the concept of a wandering uterus, I think we should pause before proclaiming that a psychiatric disorder is tied to a pending uterine event. For this reason, I favor a nonetiological title such as 'cyclic dysphoric disorder' or the placement of this disorder in the appendix of DSM-III-R. (Peele 1986: 1351)

Not every participant agreed with the importance of these professional disputes between gynecologists and psychiatrists. According to Severino, the dispute between psychiatrists and gynecologists was overstated. In trying to downplay the conflict, she points to the changing name of the diagnosis as a result of psychiatrists' collaboration with obstetricians and gynecologists. The name shift from Periluteal Phase Dysphoric Disorder to Late Luteal Phase Dysphoric Disorder came from a Washington, D.C. meeting on December 4, 1986 of the Health Care Commission of The American College of Obstetricians and Gynecologists (Severino, personal interview, May 24, 1991).

Cooperation and even consultation with gynecologists were emphasized by other participants wishing to blunt professional antagonisms. In public explanations of the name change, the increased specificity and exactness implied by the new name were emphasized. For example, in the Spitzer et. al. article in the *American Journal of Psychiatry* describing the diagnosis of LLPDD, the following explanation was given:

> Months later, in recognition of the small number of cases that occur in women who are not menstruating, the name was changed to 'periluteal phase dysphoric disorder.' The name was later changed once again, when as a result of a dialogue with colleagues from obstetrics and gynecology, it was recognized that, strictly speaking, the symptoms were not 'around' ("peri') the luteal phase but actually occurred during the late luteal phase. (Spitzer et al. 1989:893)

COOPERATION OR CONTINUED CONFLICT?

In official and semiofficial accounts of the controversy, cooperation of the professions of gynecology and psychiatry is lauded. The professional division of labor in medicine seems clear and free of conflict. However, divisions between the two medical specialties over PMS and LLPDD were still unresolved. To judge from a medical textbook on obstetrics and gynecology published just after the LLPDD controversy, the division of labor between psychiatrists and gynecologists in the treatment of PMS is still ambiguous. The authors write that when women first seek help from a physician, they frequently "inform the doctor that they are 'going crazy'" (Wilson and Carrington 1987:119). They go on to conclude that "Once symptoms characterizing PMS are identified, the patient should be reassured that she is not becoming psychotic and that there are measures that can be taken to help her" (1987:119). Medical measures given as examples of appropriate treatment include keeping a daily diary of symptoms and behaviors, exercise and dietary changes, diuretics, oral contraceptives, and antidepressants (1987). However, in what is portrayed as a rare event, those women with "marked alteration in mood swings with manic and/or severe depressive symptoms, as well as those

exhibiting psychotic behavior, should have a psychiatric evaluation before treatment" (1987:120).

This "convenient" and "public" division of labor between the gynecologic and psychiatric symptoms and treatments is further supported for
other nonmedical reasons as outlined by Robert Reid, one of the leading
gynecologists in the PMS field:

> For example, when a gynecologist is confronted by a patient who relates a
> history of severe cyclic depression in relation to menstruation in the mid-
> dle of a busy clinic, options for intervention may seem very limited. The gy-
> necologist may . . . out of frustration and perhaps fear of litigation if the
> interdisciplinary boundary that separates gynecology from psychiatry is
> transgressed choose to refer the patient to a psychiatric colleague. (Reid
> 1986:924)

But Reid goes on to warn doctors that this option could reinforce women's
fear of "going crazy" and "unless the psychiatrist is 'tuned in' to menstrual cycle-related illness, may result in a long series of unsuccessful psychiatric interventions at times with inappropriate labeling of the patient as a
manic depressive" (Reid 1986:924).

On the other side of the professional fence, psychiatrist Roger Fink,
M.D. (who served as Co-Chair of the Ad Hoc Committee that evaluated
LLPDD in 1985–1986) was concerned about how gynecologists (lumped
together with obstetricians or OB/GYNs) mistreat women with PMS. He
wrote the following when he was President-elect of the APA:

> The real question that we have to face is what percentage of the population
> is not getting adequate treatment because an obstetrician tries to handle this
> with hormonal replacement or other kinds of treatments that are not ad-
> dressing the psychological-behavioral symptomatology. (as found in *Psychi-
> atric News*, December 4, 1987)

In spite of continued wariness on the part of both medical specialties, the
effect remained the same. Psychiatrists were able to change the code number of LLPDD and to claim the psychological elements of PMS as part of
their professional province. In this way, they avoided any further *public*
conflict with gynecologists. PMS as found in LLPDD could and should be
diagnosed by a psychiatrist. PMS as a gynecological condition could still
remain the treatment province of the gynecologist. However, the differential ability to distinguish between them lies in the psychiatric province.

Additionally, in spite of what gynecologists might have thought about
the creation of this disorder and its separate code number, the power to create and classify psychiatric disorders ultimately rests with the APA. The
APA chose to reinforce the division of labor within the medical profession

by claiming jurisdictional control over the right to diagnose and treat the emotional and psychological disturbances of PMS. Through its name, code number, and distinctively psychiatric symptomatology, Late Luteal Phase Dysphoric Disorder began to establish a difference between the psychiatric and gynecologic claims to PMS—separate but equal spheres of diagnosis and practice.

INTERNAL DISPUTES AND THE PUBLIC IMAGE OF PSYCHIATRISTS

Within the psychiatric profession, practitioners debated competing paradigms of methodological and theoretical perspectives. The DSM-III revisions, and its controversial diagnoses, provided an occasion in which these disputes were played out. During the controversy, the public image of psychiatrists fighting among each other (and with other mental health professionals) was perceived as a threat to the authority and credibility of the profession. This section addresses these internal disputes among psychiatrists and how psychiatrists tried to limit the damage done to their professional image.

As one of three controversial diagnoses specifically related to women, Premenstrual Dysphoric Disorder (LLPDD) was often linked or compared to the proposed Masochistic Personality Disorder (which later was renamed Self Defeating Personality Disorder) and Paraphilic Rapism (later Coercive) Disorder. One charge leveled against APA leaders suggested that they were unwilling to change views grounded in "psychoanalytic anecdotes," not scientific research (Goleman 1985). "Their diagnoses tend to represent one narrow orientation—psychoanalytic—and one profession—psychiatry" charged then-President of the Feminist Therapy Institute (found in Holden 1986). The irony of this statement is that the DSM-III-R and LLPDD are considered a *rejection* of the influence of psychoanalytic theory—although the suggested inclusion for Masochistic Personality Disorder did come from the psychoanalytic corner of the psychiatric profession.[14]

Although a psychoanalytic theory of PMS was developed at the time Frank (1931) described it as a neurological problem, psychoanalysts have not dealt much with PMS. However, in the same year that Frank was claiming PMS for gynecologists, noted psychoanalyst Karen Horney suggested that PMS was the result of unresolved tensions within a woman about having children (Horney 1931). But nothing much came from Horney's speculation. Instead, LLPDD developed from the efforts to create a more scientific and systematic definition for PMS. Scientific research on PMS and LLPDD now relates primarily to the hormone system and brain, not the unconscious mind or the uterus. This move toward biological descriptions of PMS is consistent with the general movement toward medical and biological classifications of all mental disorders.

As argued in Chapter 2, the psychoanalytic perspective has held a strong influence on American psychiatry for a major portion of this century, especially since World War II. However, nonpsychoanalytic paradigms such as biological psychiatry have become successful and heavily influenced the definition and treatment of the mentally ill. The development of DSM-III and DSM-III-R has been especially important for the shifting nature of psychiatry as a profession.

Disputes among psychoanalysts and biologically driven psychiatrists were important for the debate over LLPDD. There appeared to be some effort to please psychoanalysts by including masochistic personality disorder in DSM-III-R. However, the association of LLPDD with the masochistic personality disorder was distorted in public debates. This troubled some psychiatrists, who believed that the image of psychiatry as science and as a medical profession was damaged.

Paul Chodoff, a psychoanalyst involved in the revision the DSM, commented in 1986 that psychodynamically oriented psychiatrists in private practice generally hold DSM-III in low regard (and DSM-III-R as well). In spite of this, he called on psychoanalysts and psychotherapists "to contain their impatience" and to use the product (DSM-III-R) (1986:203). Chodoff's exhortation for psychoanalysts to stay within the profession of medicine and psychiatry is voiced by other psychiatrists concerned about their public image.

The public image of psychiatry is as salient for the American Psychiatric Association as it is for any other professional organization. The antipsychiatry and labeling movement in the 1960s and 1970s caused public image problems for psychiatrists (see Chapter 2). The controversy over the deletion of homosexuality from DSM-II (see Bayer 1987), and the internal battle with psychoanalysts over DSM-III (Millon 1986), did not help the "scientific" or medical image of psychiatry and psychiatrists. As it happens, during the LLPDD controversy, the APA was already conducting a massive public relations campaign to improve its image (see Pasnau 1986, 1987). Roger Peele rather understated the point when he wrote: "[t]hese controversies have not enhanced the credibility of psychiatric knowledge" (1986: 1348). In letters written to officers of the APA during the controversy, psychiatrists voiced similar concerns about the public image of the profession:

> The public is watching and very much involved. The content of the DSM and the procedures we use to establish its content, are watched with a rapacious curiosity. I find this volume to be very useful and informative, but its process

and content go to the very heart of psychiatric credibility and scientific approach. (letter to Robert Pasnau, November 22, 1985)[15]

Another psychiatrist stated that the new controversial categories "may well be embarrassing to Psychiatry as a whole" (letter to Paul Fink, June 19, 1986).[16] And from a member of the Assembly of District Branches:

> I think that if published as it is revised it would ruin psychiatrists' credibility, it would be detrimental for the Association's public image and would further distance the psychiatrists from other medical specialties and from their patients. (letter to Robert Pasnau, November 20, 1985)[17]

This concern for adverse publicity was echoed in the anonymous psychiatrist's comment first quoted in Chapter 4 that "The Board of Trustees seems to have an unerring instinct for public relations fiascoes and self-destructive, ambivalent obsessions. This mess doesn't help psychiatry at all" (as quoted in *The Psychiatric Times*, August, 1986).

But this belief was not shared by Robert Spitzer, who believes instead that controversy is good for the advancement of scientific knowledge—about LLPDD and other psychiatric diagnoses. When asked how he felt about the controversy over inclusion of LLPDD, Spitzer stated:

> I mean it was a challenge. It [LLPDD] was only one front of many that I was dealing with, but . . . that was the job. I enjoy controversy. I love it, so. . . . And I loved this diagnosis more than the others. I mean, I think it has more to argue for it than the others that were controversial. (personal interview, May 23, 1991)

Although Spitzer believes that controversy is an enjoyable challenge, the tenor of the debate—and responses by the Board of Trustees to LLPDD and other diagnoses—was perceived as a threat to the scientific integrity and mission of psychiatry. Spitzer said as much in his interview with me in May 1991: "I think scientists should do what they need to do and if there's controversy, you face it. You don't try to avoid controversy" (personal interview, May 23, 1991). Spitzer believes that the Board of Trustees yielded to the special interests of the Women's Committee and ignored or didn't support their own scientific advisors:

> Now, if the Board of Trustees . . . I mean it's interesting, what would've happened. Supposed the Board of Trustees said: 'Gee, we're not going to second guess Bob Spitzer,' you know. 'We'll go with it. Let the feminists scream bloody murder.' What would've happened? There was nothing they [the opponents] could've done. I supposed they could've had a referendum but that's not the way the Board of Trustees work. The Board of Trustees is com-

prised to do something that it thinks its membership will be most comfortable with. (personal interview, May 23, 1991)

Because of this internal opposition to LLPDD, Spitzer stated that the Board of Trustees "had to do what they did" because they are "comprised to do something that it thinks it membership will be most comfortable with. And I think the membership is probably most comfortable with it [the inclusion of LLPDD in the appendix]." He stated further that "[y]ou're not going to have the Board of Trustees infuriate their own . . . you're just not going to have it. There's no way. The Board of Trustees, for years has been bending over backward to minority groups and gays" (personal interview, May 23, 1991).

In spite of professional interest in maintaining a positive public image for psychiatry, numerous groups within psychiatry made formal and public objections to the inclusion of LLPDD. These included the APA Committee on Women, the Association of Gay and Lesbian Psychiatrists, the Association of Women Psychiatrists, the Canadian Psychiatric Association Section of Women's Issues in Psychiatry, and individual psychiatrists in the Coalition Against Misdiagnosis, the Feminist Therapy Institute, the National Coalition for Women's Mental Health (see Figure 5.1).

A positive public image of psychiatry was an issue of professional importance for these groups. However, the public voicing of their objections to the stigmatization of women or other minority groups was *more important*. These groups within the profession of psychiatry saw the inclusion of LLPDD (and other controversial diagnoses) to be equally harmful (as the controversy itself). A public image of psychiatry that labels and stigmatizes women's bodies and minds as mental illness was undesirable both for political and professional reasons.

INTERPROFESSIONAL DISPUTES

The third dispute in this domain involves groups *external* to the psychiatric profession who have long engaged the APA in lengthy boundary disputes over the treatment and definition of mental illness. These include psychologists, social workers, and psychiatric nurses. The importance of the diagnostic manual in demarcating professional boundaries, expertise, and authority is highlighted by the DSM revision process. According to sociologist Phil Brown:

[f]or professional groups, diagnosis functions to define, demarcate, and develop the profession. It is a major organizing feature of the profession, as evidenced in writings by the formulators and supporters of the American Psychiatric Association. (1987:43)

Figure 5.1. Mental health organizations against the inclusion of LLPDD in the DSM-III-R

Groups Within the Psychiatric Profession

American Psychiatric Association Committee on Women
Association of Gay and Lesbian Psychiatrists
Association of Women Psychiatrists
Canadian Psychiatric Association Section of Women's Issues in Psychiatry

Groups External to the American Psychiatric Association

American Orthopsychiatric Association
American Orthopsychiatric Association Women's Study Group
American Psychological Association
American Psychological Association, Committee on Women
American Psychological Association, Division of School Psychology
American Psychological Association, Division of Counseling Psychology
Association for Women in Psychology
Canadian Psychological Association
Coalition Against Misdiagnosis
Feminist Therapy Institute
National Association of Social Workers
National Association of Social Workers: Committee on Women's Issues
National Coalition for Women's Mental Health
New Jersey Psychological Association
New York State Psychological Association: Division of Women's Issues
Network of Clinical Specialists in Mental Health/Psychiatric Nursing
Women's Special Interest Group (the Association for the Advancement of
    Behavior Therapy)

Note: I based this list upon letters of protest written in the name of the organization to the American Psychiatric Association or upon public press statements by spokespersons for the organizations.

By the end of the debate over the DSM-III-R, all major mental health associations outside of the American Psychiatric Association had gone on public record in opposition to inclusion of LLPDD (also found in Figure 5.1).

The DSM-III-R is the property and official statement of the APA; as such, it is formally recognized as the means to code and reimburse mental health care. Other mental health workers are thus "forced" to use it. This puts the APA in an organizational and structural position of power within the mental health hierarchy. Given that the more "medical" model of PMS was legitimated in LLPDD and emphasized in DSM-III-R, it would follow that psychiatrists—and not psychologists or other mental health practitioners—would define and treat PMS as a mental "illness." In constructing LLPDD as a psychiatric disorder, psychiatrists were seen by other mental health professionals as asserting their professional dominance and control of the diagnostic process—claiming a special ability to deal with PMS as a biological and psychiatric phenomenon.

At the core of this debate was a concern that psychiatrists are biased in favor of individually centered perspectives on the physiological, chemical, or biological natures of mental illness. Because of this, they may fail to consider fully social and environmental influences upon human behavior. Psychiatrists are pictured as proponents of the medical model of mental illness, which excludes or denigrates the skills and perspectives of other practitioners in the mental health hierarchy. According to Klerman, the term "medical model" means different things to different professions: "[t]o psychologists and social workers in mental health settings, it is a term of contempt to use in the struggle over whether medical degrees are necessary for positions of greater authority or higher salary" (1977:221).

Underlying the debate was a practical issue surrounding use of the DSM-III-R. The majority of psychologists and social workers are required to use the DSM-III-R diagnoses for coding patients in organizational contexts and/or for the third-party reimbursement for psychotherapy. According to two major critics of the DSM from social work:

> Probably the greatest stimulus to the renaissance of psychiatric diagnosis has been the expansion of third-party reimbursement for psychotherapy through private health insurance, employee assistance programs, and services for the medically indigent. These programs usually require a diagnosis, and DSM-III is often the designated reference cited. It must be used even by therapists who doubt the value of formal diagnosis. In surveys, a majority of psychologists and social workers say that they use DSM only because it is required. (Kutchins and Kirk 1988:6)

This was hardly a new issue. In 1976, psychiatrists and psychologists attempted to define a mental disorder in the Work Group to Revise DSM-II. Two members of the DSM-III Work Group, Robert Spitzer and his colleague Jean Endicott (a psychologist), developed a definition of a mental disorder as "a subset of medical disorders" (see Millon 1986; Spitzer et al. 1980). This "led to a bitter exchange of letters with the American Psychological Association, which challenged the basis for designating the DSM-III disorders as 'medical'" (Spitzer et al. 1980).

Blashfield has pointed out that such jurisdictional disputes create trouble for a medical model of psychiatry (1984:80). Two psychologists noted the jurisdictional issues related to these professional boundaries 15 years ago:

> It is entirely possible, for example, that promulgation of DSM-III as an official action of the American Psychiatric Association will carry sufficient weight to call it to the attention of insurers and legislators who will see it in quasi-official recognition of the primacy of physicians in the diagnosis and

treatment of the disorders categorized by DSM-III. Since these disorders are inclusive of virtually every psychological ill to which men and women are heir, little will be left for psychologists and other mental health professionals to work with. Even less will be left if legislators and third-party payers conclude that, since these conditions are all 'medical disorders,' they must first be evaluated by physicians, who will then decide whether they or ancillary mental health professionals (e.g., the psychologists) will treat the disorder. (Schact and Nathan 1977:1024)

The idea that mental disorders are a subset of *medical* disorders was brought up in the DSM-III-R controversy, but did not take on the same meaning as before. Robert Spitzer argued before the Board of Trustees at their June 1986 meeting (which decided the placement of LLPDD in the appendix) "that the Board should 'face up to the issue of what is a mental disorder,' which he described as a medical disorder presenting primarily with mental or behavior symptoms" (as quoted in *Psychiatric News*, July 18, 1986:7).

What is really interesting in the conflict between psychiatrists and other mental health workers is that the rhetoric of opposition statements among nonpsychiatric professions within the mental field took a different tactic than in earlier DSM confrontations. The supporting statements of the professional associations adhered to and supported the claims of the psychiatric association's own Committee on Women about the lack of scientific evidence and the possible stigmatization effect of LLPDD. The focus on "science" and "stigmatization" served to deflect public criticism that their opposition was "purely" professional in nature. No explicit mention of *control* by the psychiatric profession was contained in any of the "official" statements about LLPDD by other mental health organizations.

The list of mental-health organizations and the number of psychologists and social workers who individually wrote letters of protest to the American Psychiatric Association opposing inclusion were substantial. A resolution passed by the American Psychological Association's Board of Directors charged that the psychiatric association had developed the diagnosis "without presenting any adequate scientific basis" and called the diagnosis "potentially dangerous to women" (Adler 1990b:12). Primary opposition came from the Committee on Women in Psychology, which worked closely with the Committee on Women of the psychiatric association. The Psychological Association focused on the potential harm to women, and did not make any explicit statement about professional boundaries. A statement from the American Psychological Association's Committee on Women emphasized that "We feel that the diagnosis has ominous implications for perpetuating damaging stereotypes of women and for fostering an unnecessarily pathological view of women's experience" (letter to Robert Spitzer, dated September 16, 1985).

The National Association of Social Workers (NASW) statement came much later in the controversy (May 1986). As Kutchins and Kirk indicated, "[t]he strong reaction from social workers was unanticipated because not a single critical article about DSM-III had appeared in a social work journal before the statement was released" (Kutchins and Kirk 1989a:94). Social workers constitute the largest professional group in the mental health field, and also use the DSM more frequently than any other diagnostic reference book (see Kirk and Kutchins 1992). Therefore, public opposition by the NASW, which involved an intensive writing campaign objecting to inclusion of LLPDD and supporting an NASW liaison to the DSM revision process, was nothing to be taken lightly. The NASW statement read:

> While social workers recognize that women do experience cycle-related changes, we are disturbed by the vague and over-general nature of the diagnostic criteria for this proposed diagnosis, and foresee its serious abuse in the current political climate. (Position statement on 3-R by NASW, dated May 31, 1986)[18]

The Organization for Obstetric, Gynecologic & Neonatal Nurses (NAACOG) also wrote a formal letter of protest, in support of the APA Committee on Women:

> Clearly, there are needs for greater data and research on PMS. Rigorous study should be undertaken to define the syndrome with more accuracy. Clearer definitions are needed in regard to the hormonal, behavioral, and psychiatric changes that are exhibited. These clear definitions still elude us. Much more study and research data are needed. (letter dated August 29, 1985)[19]

The construction of the psychiatric diagnosis of LLPDD ultimately signified the addition of more mental health "professional turf" for psychiatrists. Opposition by nonpsychiatric professions to inclusion of LLPDD did help put the diagnosis in the appendix rather than the main text of the manual. However, the professionally related argument that PMS has social, economic, and interpersonal bases was not explicitly acknowledged—but neither were the claims rejected—when the Board of Trustees voted to place the diagnosis related to PMS in the appendix of DSM-III-R.

That LLPDD was placed in the *appendix* (and not in the main text) is a measure of the extent to which the leaders of the American Psychiatric Association were "mindful" of angered opposition from other mental health professionals. The influence of nonpsychiatric professions in the mental health field was not ignored. This is underscored during Robert Pasnau's term of office as president of the APA from 1986 to 1987. The APA became active in outreach programs to psychology, social work, and nursing. He addressed the Board of Directors of the NASW and participated in a conference of the Joint Commission on Interprofessional Affairs. In his Presidential address to the APA, Pasnau clearly stated his intentions:

During our present remedicalization we cannot, on behalf of our patients, turn our backs on colleagues in allied mental health disciplines. . . . All of the professions recognize the potential for benefit though collaboration, both to the professions and to our patients. We believe that when spokespersons of our four professions publicly disparage the competency and ethics of the others' professions, all of us are injured. We must do all we can to eliminate unnecessary tension between us while we continue to articulate our special areas of competency. This is sometimes a delicate balance. (Pasnau 1987:978)

The opposition to the inclusion of LLPDD by the nonpsychiatric mental health professions was defeated with the inclusion of the diagnosis in the manual—even with its placement in the appendix. The argument that PMS has social, economic, and interpersonal bases in reality was not upheld in the settlement. The construction of the psychiatric diagnosis of LLPDD signified the addition of more mental health "professional turf" for psychiatrists. However, other mental health professionals were successful in one aspect as a result of their opposition to DSM-III-R revisions.

As a result of their opposition to the DSM-III-R revisions, psychologists, social workers, and psychiatric nurses made some professional gains. As sociologist Donald Light observed recently, the mental health care domain exhibits "the largest and most successful turf battle in the past 25 years" by psychologists and social workers (Light 1988:207). DSM-IV proceeded with formal liaisons with the American Psychological Association, the National Association of Social Workers, and other health and mental health organizations. As a "mid-term" report on the DSM-IV development stated:

The task force has also established formal liaisons with the American Psychological Association, the American Psychological Society, the National Association of Social Workers, the American Nursing Association, the American Occupational Therapy Association, and over 60 additional organizations and associations interested in the development of DSM-IV. (Frances, et al. 1990:1442)

As a result of the DSM-III-R controversies, the APA tried to reduce interprofessional conflict over the DSM-IV.

GROUPS OUTSIDE THE HEALTH AND MENTAL HEALTH PROFESSIONS

The final issue in this domain concerns the role of semiprofessional, self-help, and nontraditional healers in treating and diagnosing PMS. This boundary-conflict was less visible than the others, but was significant nevertheless. Was PMS to be diagnosed and treated by a doctor, a psychiatrist, or a mental health professional, or by alternative healers (including the patient herself). The demarcation of PMS as a mental versus a physical disorder was significant not just to gynecologists and psychiatrists, but also to advocates of self-help treatments and to the pharmaceutical industry.

As discussed in Chapter 1, increased public awareness of PMS resulted in a rise in the number of self-help books (e.g., Wade 1984; Kass-Annese and Danzer 1987; Bender 1989) and PMS treatment clinics (such as the PMS Action, Inc. in Irvine, California). Over-the-counter PMS tablets, self-help books, and PMS advice articles that focus upon diet, stress, and exercise have all become big business since the 1980s. For example, in *PMS: Questions and Answers*, the charting of symptoms is described as "the most effective, least expensive way to determine if you have PMS" (Bender 1989:4). Although professional and medical options are presented, reliance upon the self and other support systems such as family and friends is encouraged. For example, in response to the question of "Can my family doctor be my PMS doctor?" Bender gives the following answer:

> I would have to answer with a qualified yes. If your physician seems knowledgeable and demonstrates a genuine concern for the problem, listen carefully. At the same time, do some of your own research by reading the published information on PMS and talking to other individuals who have the syndrome. Be willing to express your own ideas on PMS to your health care practitioner. The end result should be an effective team effort. If you are dissatisfied with your doctor's approach, you have the option of seeking a second or third opinion. Trust yourself and your instincts. If the doctor you see first doesn't feel right, don't be afraid to look elsewhere. (Bender 1989:138–139)

On the other hand, a gynecologist treating patients with PMS wrote that "a medical problem of major proportion may be obscured by the patient's interpretation of her own symptoms" as PMS (Vigliani 1988:182). An editorial in *The New England Journal of Medicine* expressed fear that "many women are so desperate that they will seek out any form of therapy. Unfortunately, that has resulted in the development of clinics specializing in premenstrual syndrome, which are being merchandized like many of the fast-food chains. Such clinics frequently provide unproved or ineffective forms of therapy" (Vaitukaitis 1984:1372) (see Chapter 7 for more discussion of scientific treatments and practitioners).

Concern over nonprofessional treatments of PMS arose early in the debate over LLPDD. Challenges to the professional expertise of psychiatry were so significant that Spitzer explicitly stated:

When psychiatry is under attack, you must not equivocate. There is no doubt that what we call periluteal phase dysphoric disorder (the newly adopted name for what had been called premenstrual dysphoric disorder) exists as a clinically significant syndrome in some women, even though the causes and optimal therapy are unknown. We must call this a mental disorder! (*The Psychiatric Times*, August 1986)

The reasoning goes: if PMS as manifested in LLPDD is seen only as a mental disorder, the physical or gynecological symptoms are downplayed and women would by-pass alternative and self-help treatments. In the first few months of the controversy, Spitzer was concerned about "a large number of semiprofessional groups treating this condition," which he stated "need a psychiatrist's skill" (*Psychiatric News*, October 18, 1985:6). As indicated in Chapter 3, physical symptoms were added to the list of criteria for an LLPDD diagnosis at the dictate of the Ad Hoc Committee in December 1985. This move was done to satisfy women's health and feminist critics, who didn't want the diagnosis to suggest that PMS is all in women's "heads." But this move also claimed jurisdictional boundaries for the treatment of disorders by the psychiatric profession. According to Roger Peele of the Work Group and the Ad Hoc Committee:

To remove it [PDD] completely from DSM-III-R is unattractive, however, because thousands of people are self-diagnosing and self-medicating themselves as though they have premenstrual dysphoric disorder and are otherwise going untreated. We want these people to see psychiatrists since, among other reasons, studies have shown that many such self-diagnosed patients do not have a cyclic disorder but have another psychiatric disorder. (Peele 1986:1351)

This issue of professional jurisdiction in the diagnosis and treatment of mental disorders is also highlighted by a "cautionary statement" printed near the front of the DSM-III-R, which states:

The specified diagnostic criteria for each mental disorder are offered as guidelines for making diagnoses, since it has been demonstrated that the use of such criteria enhances agreement among clinicians and investigators. The proper use of these criteria requires specialized clinical training that provides both a body of knowledge and clinical skills. (American Psychiatric Association 1987:xxix)

An example of one of these challenges to psychiatry is found in an advertisement one drug company ran in *People* magazine in the week in which the Board of Trustees made their decision about the PMS diagnosis in June 1986. The two-page ad was from Chattem Pharmaceutical, which produces an over-the-counter PMS drug called PreMysyn PMS (see the advertisement in *People* Weekly for June 30, 1986). The graphic image of the psychiatric couch with medical diplomas hanging on the wall is accompanied by the headline "Premenstrual Tension is not something to take lying down." The subtext goes on to explain that premenstrual tension is "not a psychological issue. It is a physical condition." This advertisement tells women to "use their head" so that this product can get "to the physical source of Premenstrual Tension." Self-medication is empowerment yet safe since it comes with recommendations from "leading OB/GYNS." It is this type of challenge to the professional expertise of psychiatrists (and upholding the expertise of gynecologists) that lies at the heart of professional dominance issues.

The challenge to the expertise of health and mental health professions also overlaps the rise of the women's health movement and the resurgence of a feminist movement in the 1970s. As a result of these interrelated movements, women challenged the expertise of professionals to define and treat conditions or disorders related to women's bodies. As such, this challenge overlaps and leads into the feminist debate about the definition, treatment, and control of women's health and illness experiences. This explicitly feminist and gendered challenge to the psychiatric profession moves the analysis into the woman domain (Chapter 6).

CONCLUSION

In the Health and Mental Health Domain, I have established that LLPDD—as constituted both by sociological literature and by actors involved in the controversy—was the site of professional competition for dominance in the health and mental health fields. I have demonstrated this by examining four major conflicts among health and mental health providers. First, LLPDD was the result of gynecologists' and psychiatrists' struggle to define PMS as differentially physical and mental. Second, within competing schools or perspectives within psychiatry, LLPDD is seen as a product or result of the increasing biologization of psychiatric diagnosis and the rise in neo-Kraepelinian thought. The third conflict over LLPDD came between competing professional and therapeutic groups, such as psychologists, social workers, and psychiatric nurses, in the debate over the social and economic bases of LLPDD and other defined mental disorders. The final challenge came from self-help and providers of over-the-counter medication, who also claimed a right to define and treat PMS.

In each conflict in this domain, LLPDD was shaped by controversy over the right to define, diagnose, and treat mental conditions. In constructing PMS as a psychiatric disorder, the APA was also successful in extending its professional boundaries on three fronts and in redefining its own professional mission within the psychiatric profession.

NOTES

1. The relationship of ICD-9-CM to DSM-III-R is explained further in Chapter 3.
2. Found at the American Psychiatric Association Archives, Washington, D.C.
3. Found at the American Psychiatric Association Archives, Washington, D.C.
4. Found at the American Psychiatric Association Archives, Washington, D.C.
5. Found at the American Psychiatric Association Archives, Washington, D.C.
6. Found at the American Psychiatric Association Archives, Washington, D.C.
7. Found at the American Psychiatric Association Archives, Washington, D.C.
8. Found at the American Psychiatric Association Archives, Washington, D.C.
9. Found at the American Psychiatric Association Archives, Washington, D.C.
10. Found at the American Psychiatric Association Archives, Washington, D.C.
11. Found at the American Psychiatric Association Archives, Washington, D.C.
12. Found in the personal archives of Dr. Jean Hamilton, Institute of Research on Women's Health, Washington, D.C.
13. Found at the American Psychiatric Association Archives, Washington, D.C.
14. The inclusion of Masochistic Personality Disorder was seen by some as a way to mollify the psychoanalysts in the profession.
15. Found at the American Psychiatric Association Archives, Washington, D.C.
16. Found at the American Psychiatric Association Archives, Washington, D.C.
17. Found at the American Psychiatric Association Archives, Washington, D.C.
18. Found at the American Psychiatric Association Archives, Washington, D.C.
19. Found at the American Psychiatric Association Archives, Washington, D.C.

6

Who Defines a Normal and Healthy Woman?: The Woman Domain

[Women] are particularly irate at the way they are treated by gynecologists. These women dislike being denied the right to participate fully in decisions about their bodies. They are particularly bitter that they are ignorant and incompetent to do this because doctors make it difficult for them to acquire the information they need to make competent decisions for themselves. (Ruzek 1981:563–564)

Early public accounts of the battle over LLPDD clearly identified it as a "woman's or feminist issue" (see Chapter 4 for a discussion of the various accounts). "Feminists," it was said, were upset over the possibility of stigmatization from inclusion of a psychiatric diagnosis in DSM-III-R that affects only women. This representation of LLPDD as a "woman's issue" clearly identifies the existence of a woman domain and the need for its analysis. However, as the above statement by women's health analyst Sheryl Ruzek suggests, (written before the controversy began in 1983), other less-obviously gendered issues are involved in the issue of women's health. How and why a controversial scientific or technical artifact is called a "woman's issue" is important for understanding the gendered nature of scientific diagnoses and medical treatments. Who defines and treats women and their bodies? Do women have a say? How can women more fully participate in their health and medical care?

Arguments constructed in the feminist and women's health literatures influenced the nature of the debate and the constitution of LLPDD as an artifact of the woman domain. I begin by showing how and why the rhetoric of the feminist and women's health movement articulated strategies of actors opposed to the inclusion of LLPDD, on grounds of the dangers of growing medicalization and of the stigmatization of psychiatric diagnoses related to women. This is followed by specific examination of the controversy in the context of the three gendered ownership claims. Professional women claimed expertise to speak for all women, and some individual women claimed expertise to speak for themselves about PMS. The ownership claims drew upon the rhetorical tactics and political positions from the women's health and feminist literatures.

FEMINISM AND THE WOMEN'S HEALTH MOVEMENT

For the past 30 years, the feminist movement and feminist scholarship have been major influences in identifying and defining important social, political, and economic issues pertaining to women. Raising the "consciousness" of women to be aware of their health and their bodies has been one of its primary goals. The rise of a feminist and women-centered scholarship in academic and wider communities in the 1970s has provided the greatest source of material about women's health (Ruzek 1978; Corea [1975] 1985). As Riessman points out, feminist critics

> have been important voices in changing women's consciousness about their health. They have identified the sexual politics embedded in conceptions of sickness and beliefs about appropriate care. In addition, they have provided the analytic basis for a social movement that has as its primary goal the reclaiming of knowledge about and control over women's bodies. (1983:3)

Writers, workers, and supporters of the feminist movement, and, in particular, the women's health movement, are seen as advocates and defenders of better health and medical care for all women.

Ehrenreich and English's work is among the most important feminist health writings that emerged from the resurgent American women's movement in the early 1970s. *For Her Own Good: 150 Years of the Expert's Advice to Women* (1978) is a commonly cited work on women and health. Here and elsewhere (1973a,b), Ehrenreich and English argue that the rise of the male medical profession has been deleterious for women's physical health and mental health. The gendered state of relations between male experts and women patients is said to be the cause:

> The experts wooed their female constituency, promising the 'right' and scientific way to live, and women responded—most eagerly in the upper and middle classes, more slowly among the poor—with dependency and trust. It was never an equal relationship, for the experts' authority rested on the denial or destruction of women's autonomous sources of knowledge: the old networks of skill-sharing, the accumulated lore of generations of mothers. (Ehrenreich and English 1978: 4–5)

Although there has been criticism of their scholarship, Ehrenreich and English provided a spur to the women's self-help movement. More academic and empirically grounded analyses of the gendered nature of medical and scientific knowledge have followed.[1]

At a more practical or experiential level, the women's health movement helped educate women about their bodies, and advocated reform from within as well as outside conventional medical worlds (Todd 1989). The women's self help and clinic movement (as exemplified in The National Women's Health Network) has been responsible for the spread of medical information and the self-education of women through newsletters and in self-help medical books (Ruzek 1978). Organizations such as the Boston Women's Health Collective have provided women with access to information about their bodies and treatments of it by the medical profession, in books such as *Our Bodies, Ourselves* (1973) and *The New Our Bodies, Ourselves* ([1984] 1992a).

The women's health movement has also found allies within the academic world. Scholarly research has burgeoned on issues related to women's history, women's bodies, and the women's health movement (Scully and Bart 1973; Ruzek 1978; Fee 1983; Jacobus et al. 1990; Hubbard 1990). A central theme in these academic studies has focused upon the process of medicalization. The definition of "medicalization" comes from medical sociology, but it has been particularly useful for feminist analysts to describe the relationship between women and the usually male, medical profession (Riessman 1983:3).

Medicalization is the expansion of medicine as a major institution of social control in society (Friedson 1970a; Zola 1972), and particularly in areas traditionally viewed in moral or religious terms (Conrad and Schneider 1980; Tomes 1990). According to Reissman (1983), medicalization is composed of two interrelated social processes: (1) a medical meaning is given to a behavior or condition, and (2) medicine is responsible for eliminating or controlling behaviors and experiences defined as deviant.

Women have played an important role in their own medicalization process. Riessman makes a strong argument that women have not been passive "victims" in the medicalization process. PMS is often used as a current example of women giving medicalized accounts of their own situations, and holding out for the possibility of medical help or cures (Riessman 1983). To the question "why do women act out in rage or emotional responses to life situations?" a scientific-medical answer says that these women are suffering from PMS and cannot help the hormonal imbalance in their bodies. Who can "help" women control themselves? Help can come only from medical doctors, psychiatrists, or scientists who "understand" the biological and medical basis of women's behaviors. As Susan Bell argues so forcefully:

> PMS is becoming medicalized. It is being defined as a medical problem and medical personnel are being given the responsibility for treating it. In the

process, behaviors that previously were identified as the symptoms of neurosis or criminality or the products of women's imaginations are coming to be seen as manifestations of a biological imbalance that can be diagnosed and treated by medical professionals. (Bell 1987:155)

In a society that relies heavily on the authority of scientific explanations of reality, it seems only natural that women would want scientific-medical explanations for their feelings and bodies.

In spite of the assertion that women play a collaborative role in the medicalization of female-related disorders, Riessman is quick to point out that negative social, political, and economic effects of medicalization are often severe. Riessman indicates the paradoxes:

> The medicalization of human problems is a contradictory reality for women. It is part of the problem and of the solution. It has grown out of and in turn has created a series of paradoxes. As women have tried to free themselves from the control that biological processes have had over their lives, they simultaneously have strengthened the control of a biomedical view of their experience. As women visit doctors and get symptom relief, the social causes of their problems are ignored. As doctors acknowledge women's experience and treat their problems medically, problems are stripped of their political content and popular movements are taken over. (Riessman 1983:16)

The feminist health and mental health literatures have drawn on the concept of medicalization to show how women have lost control of their bodies (and indeed of their own social movement) (Ruzek 1978; Bell 1986). For example, recent work by Emily Martin has shown how women's reproductive organs and cycles (such as PMS or menopause) have fallen under medical definition and control in late industrial societies (Martin 1987). According to Clarke, "[i]t is life-cycle events and processes, especially those involving reproductive cycles, that are typically the historically and personally significant 'moments' when medicine enters women's lives, for women's biological cycles have been profoundly medicalized" (1990a:8). This claim is supported by recent studies of medical diagnoses of hysteria, neurasthenia, menstruation, and menopause (see Bell 1986, 1987; McCrea 1983; Showalter 1985).

WOMEN AND MENTAL HEALTH

The associations of women, mental health, and menstruation have also been noticeably influential in shaping the parameters of the political and rhetorical debate about the stigmatization effects of LLPDD. Opponents argued that gender-specific mental health labels (i.e., diagnoses) adhere to rigid definitions of gender in patriarchal society and are thus harmful to women. These arguments were based upon two groundbreaking works on women and mental health published in the early 1970s. These studies informed discussions of women's mental health, and raised the stigmatization issue debated during the LLPDD controversy.

The first study consisted of mental health professionals' assessments of mentally healthy males, females, and adult persons of nonspecified sex (Broverman et al. 1970). Their study called attention to the impact of gender on professional assessments of mental health. Based on a personal inventory scale, they showed that normal healthy males were typically described as independent, logical, and adventurous. Importantly, these male-associated traits were also given as attributes of a healthy *person*. A healthy person had male characteristics. Health for a woman was portrayed in less than flattering terms. Healthy women were rated as emotional, powerless, more conceited, and dependent.[2]

Perhaps the most influential book on women and mental health is Phyllis Chesler's *Women and Madness* (1972 and 1989, second edition). Chesler states that she wrote the book in response to the growing women's health movement. She hoped to make people aware of the way women's mental health had been historically and contemporarily described (1989). She portrays a medical and psychiatric profession not only unresponsive to special needs of women's mental health, but also one that is damaging and harmful to all women in their assumption of passively gendered female characteristics.

The "Cheslerian Thesis" asserts that a sexist society makes women prone to mental illness and more likely to be committed to mental institutions (see Tomes 1990:144). Chesler concludes that there is "A double standard of mental health—and humanity—one for women, another for men, seems to good-naturedly and unscientifically dominate most theories—and treatments—of women and men" [1989 (1972):xxxv]. In a review of studies on women and mental health since Chesler, historian Nancy Tomes states that "[r]ecent research presents a much more complex picture: women are more likely than men to report emotional distress, but they do not suffer from higher rates of severe mental illness, or psychosis; neither do women outnumber men in mental hospital admissions" (1990:145).

Recent research on gender differences in mental health point to the following conclusions: sex differences show up most strongly in disorders most sensitive to cultural and social influences (Kaplan 1983; Loring and Powell 1988); women are more likely to engage in help-seeking activity for psychological problems, but they are not more likely than men to be committed to mental hospitals (see Guttentag et al. 1980); women are more likely to interpret what they are feeling or doing as signs of illness and get labeled as sick, while men deny distress and act out behaviorally and get labeled criminal, deviant, or "bad." Tomes concludes that "the historical record supports the argument that sex-role socialization may have predisposed men and women to gender-specific reasons for and modes of expressing psychological distress" (Tomes 1990:151–152). These conclusions are important in assessing the controversy about the sex-specific political nature of LLPDD and its scientific validity.

PMS AND FEMINIST COMMUNITY

Growing awareness about PMS in lay society has increased suspicion of medical-scientific worlds among the feminist and women's health communities. As suggested in Chapter 1, PMS represents a classic stigmatization and medicalization dilemma for the feminist community. On the one hand, women's health and menstrually related issues have historically either been ignored by physicians and scientists *or* women were told that any feelings or problems "are all in their heads." On the other hand, menstrually related problems have been defined or labeled as making women "crazy" or putting them "under the control of their raging hormones."[3] The reality of PMS in the woman domain meant that either it was ignored or considered a "pseudoproblem" by doctors and scientists or it was medicalized into a biological fact, which meant the women were controlled by their hormones and by "experts."

Within the feminist and women's health community, recent recognition in the past 30 years or so that premenstrual changes are "real" and significant in women's lives is seen as "progress." However, feminist scholars have been quick to point out that PMS is explicitly linked to larger cultural, political, and economic values and systems (Martin 1987; Fausto-Sterling 1985). According to Riessman, the medicalization of PMS reinforces the connection of women's emotions with their biology, and deflects attention away from the social etiology of the condition (1983:11). How PMS is defined—and who controls or owns the diagnoses related to it—is a matter of larger social, political, and economic concern.

According to most feminist scholars, it is legitimate to acknowledge a biological basis for PMS. The broader political questions of medical treatment and management remain. For example, Zita states:

> The experience of PMS is a reality for many women, and for some women it is extreme and severe. To be told that it's 'all in your head' is both insulting and arrogant. These experiences are rooted in the body and its physiological mechanisms. However, to be told that it is due to a specific hormonal imbal-

ance that can be medically managed is often overly simplistic and dangerously premature given the state of current research. (1988:94)

The feminist acknowledgment of the biological "fact" of PMS is further supported by noted PMS researcher Randi Koeske. Koeske outlined early feminist critiques of PMS research:

Acknowledgement of biological influence in women's lives is not, per se, inconsistent with feminism. It is biomedicine's tacit assumptions about the meaning and elemental nature of biological facts which must be challenged. (Koeske 1983:2)

The paradox of acknowledging PMS as legitimate yet challenging the way in which women are treated is even greater for biomedically trained healers committed to helping women. A feminist physician who treats women with PMS wrote:

The feminist in me wishes that our biology were irrelevant. The doctor in me sees the need for recognizing and treating premenstrual symptoms. The woman in me recognizes the power of the biological forces within me, and wishes I lived in a society in which my menstrual cycle were seen as an asset, not a liability. (Michelle Harrison, as quoted from the *NWHN Newsletter*, Summer 1984:5)

LLPDD AND THREE GENDERED OWNERSHIP CLAIMS

In the woman domain, there were three ownership claims (two made for women with PMS and one made by women with PMS) that constituted and constructed LLPDD as a gendered issue, i.e., specifically focusing upon the position and image of women in society. The first claim to the ownership of PMS came from women's health and mental health groups, such as the Women's Committee of the APA and the American Psychological Association and the National Coalition for Women's Mental Health. On the basis of their training, professional work, and organizational expertise, these "professional advocates" protested the inclusion of the LLPDD diagnosis on behalf of "all women." In their view, LLPDD had the potentially negative consequence of labeling all menstruating women as psychiatrically impaired. Another claim to speak on behalf of women was made by those professional experts seeking to include LLPDD as a psychiatric disorder. Finally, individual women with PMS wanted to speak and be heard as experts about their own bodies and experiences.

ANTI-INCLUSION EXPERTS

Throughout the controversy over the inclusion of LLPDD, women's health and feminist organizations argued that the psychiatric labeling of PMS as LLPDD was politically, economically, and socially harmful to all women. Based on the nature of their research or professional training, these women considered themselves to be advocates for all women and simultaneously situated their arguments within academic and research literatures on gender, feminism, and medical or scientific work. For example, a central concern they expressed is that LLPDD had the potentially negative consequence of labeling all menstruating women as psychiatrically impaired. Negative effects were predicted in employment decisions, child custody cases, and political confirmations. There was also the assertion that the diagnosis would incriminate all women in society as susceptible to their "raging hormones" once a month. In making their judgments that the inclusion of LLPDD would be harmful, individual women scientists and professional experts were staking their own claim to the ownership of PMS.

As noted earlier in the book, the first opposition to the inclusion of LLPDD came from within the American Psychiatric Association. Members of the APA's own Committee on Women initially voiced their objections and spearheaded the fight against inclusion of it in the DSM-III-R. Much to the chagrin of the APA, the Committee on Women challenged the diagnostic process by writing memos and letters, attending meetings, and conducting public protests concerning LLPDD and two other proposed diagnoses related to women. The public statements made by the members of the Committee on Women contained an urgent and strong sense of duty and responsibility to women in society. As Teresa Bernardez, the chair of this committee, stated: "it was a clear imperative" to question inclusion of LLPDD and to bring feminist expertise into the debate (personal interview, April 20, 1990, East Lansing).

Due to the organizational nature of the APA and the DSM revision process, the Committee on Women found itself in a structural position of power and authority to fight on the behalf of all women, and especially those immediately at risk from an LLPDD diagnosis. From the first meeting of the LLPDD Advisory Committee in May 1985 until the publication of the DSM-III-R in 1987, the Committee on Women worked within the existing organizational structure of the American Psychiatric Association to fight inclusion of the diagnosis. According to Spitzer, in spite of the Committee on Women's concerns, the Work Group initially had no reason to doubt that a PMS-related diagnosis would be included in DSM-III-R (personal interview, May 23, 1991, New York City). There was some early written correspondence between Hamilton and Bernardez with Spitzer, and a gathering was arranged at the Board of Trustees meeting in September 1985 to discuss the issue.[4] However, the political effectiveness of the Committee on Women's opposition was diminished so long as it remained focused only on an internal problem to the APA.

The Committee on Women chose to go outside the organizational machinery of the APA and enlisted external allies to help fight the inclusion of the PMS diagnosis. The Committee on Women's decision to go "outside" the APA apparently was not viewed favorably by officials within the organization. A letter dated January 13, 1986 to Bernardez, from officials of the APA admonished her to continue to work within the APA to more effectively gain the changes already agreed upon (letter from Robert Pasnau and Roger Peele).[5] This admonition to stay "within the ranks" provoked discussion among the Committee on Women. In a memo dated January 28, 1986, Bernardez asked the committee: "Shall we keep our final statements confined to APA members? Shall we not share them with the women from the American Psychological Association?"[6]

However, it was precisely through the use of tactics such as enlisting allies in other fields to create a public awareness about the proposed diagnosis that opposition forces were effective in drawing public attention to women's health and mental health issues.

The Institute for Research on Women's Health in Washington, D.C. became a center of activity for the LLPDD opposition movement. As professional advocates for the health and mental health of all women, the strategy involved linking the diagnosis of LLPDD (and the other proposed controversial diagnoses) to wider scientific, economic, and political issues. Women associated with the Institute for Research on Women's Health spent several months on putting together briefing booklets and doing mailings to get the word out. Jean Hamilton, the Center's director stated:

> I also had a mailing list and ties to other organizations and advocacy groups—interdisciplinary ties. So we put out the word. Also because I'm located in Washington and because I'm feminist and have connections to other nonprofit organizations in D.C., we know lobbyists and we knew press people. . . . And those people put out the word in their newsletters or in their organizations so we had this sort of feminist networking process. So we had people writing letters and creating havoc and we had all these radio spots. And that really pissed them off—I mean it really pissed them off. I mean how dare we? (Jean Hamilton, personal interview, June 4, 1990, Washington, D.C.)

With the help of a mailing list from The National Coalition for Women's Mental Health, women associated with the Institute for Research on Women's Health spent "several months on putting together how best to present our position and then doing, you know, whatever mailings. We'd

have group meetings, three or four people would come and we'd stuff envelopes . . . we must've mailed out to five or six hundred people."[7]

Professional opponents of LLPDD remained firm in their stance that
the diagnosis was ultimately harmful for all women. In the briefing prepared by the Institute for Research on Women's Mental Health, opponents
argued that "the naming of a psychiatric diagnosis after the menstrual cycle, locates the stigma—the defect or fatal difference—within the victim,
and within the very physiology of womanhood: the processes of menstruation" (IRWH 1985).[8] In their view, LLPDD had the potentially negative consequence of labeling all menstruating women as psychiatrically
impaired.

Ownership claims made by women scientists and health professionals
suggested that they could and were working on the behalf of all women.
On the basis of their training, professional work, and organizational expertise, these "professional advocates" protested the inclusion of the
LLPDD. The limited success that the Committee on Women enjoyed in
fighting the inclusion of LLPDD (the name was changed away from Premenstrual and it was included in a research appendix and not the main
text) resulted from their efforts to link the diagnosis to women's medicalization and stigmatization—making it a matter of political and economic
concern to all women. The bases of this link is found in academic and re-
search-oriented studies on women's health and mental health. It was primarily professional advocates who placed the diagnosis of LLPDD within
this broader rhetorical framework of gender politics, health, and medical
care for women. For example, in the "Action Alert Notices" that were sent
to women and women's groups across the country by Hamilton and associates, the issue of LLPDD is placed within a larger debate about women's
health by requesting that people write to the National Institutes of Health
in support of the Public Health Service's Task Force on Women's Health
guidelines.

PROINCLUSION EXPERT CLAIMS OF SPEAKING FOR WOMEN

The second claim by experts to speak for women with PMS and indeed
all women in the LLPDD debate came from proinclusion scientists and
psychiatrists. Numerous public statements by proinclusion members of
the LLPDD Advisory Committee suggested that they well understood the
objections by feminist and women's groups—but disagreed with their
"analysis." Both rhetoric and analysis in the debate turned on what exactly constituted a feminist analysis of PMS, and who had the "right" to speak
for women with PMS.

According to Robert Spitzer, the head of the Work Group revising the

DSM, the inclusion of the LLPDD diagnosis was even more important to show that *not all women* are psychiatrically affected by PMS. He stated:

> Well, one of the main arguments against the category seems to be that we would be diagnosing all women or a very large proportion. So it was important, we felt, to develop the criteria in a way that would not happen. And we thought if we could develop a questionnaire and apply it to women at risk for the disorder and show that it was actually not common, that would be helpful. (Robert Spitzer, personal interview, May 23, 1991, New York City)

Thus, in the LLPDD debate, a key pragmatic and epistemological question was: Once PMS is defined as biologically real, are women then not in the position to be helped? Instead of stigmatizing women, proinclusion scientists argued that the diagnosis was really a good thing for women. David Rubinow, head of a PMS research laboratory at NIMH, stated that in spite of feminists' concerns about stigmatization, "this [LLPDD] is a gain for feminists." Inclusion of the diagnosis would "make it clear that the great majority of women do not suffer from 'raging hormones'" (Holden 1986:231).

In spite of these initial claims, scientists' positions or arguments on LLPDD were not sex-specific. Neither all women nor women scientists and psychiatrists agreed that the inclusion was harmful. For example, women scientists comprised the majority of the LLPDD Advisory Committee that voted in favor of the inclusion of the diagnosis. Sally Severino, a practicing psychiatrist who specifically works with women and PMS, was a leading proponent of the diagnosis. She stated that the classification of PMS in the DSM-III-R "confers a legitimacy on a syndrome historically neglected by doctors and scientists" (DePaul 1986:20).

In her work as a psychiatrist, Severino stated that she had at first dismissed the notion of PMS as "real," but became convinced of the reality of the disorder after coming into contact with someone who had it. This spurred her to conduct research on PMS. She became convinced that PMS was a distinct disorder because she could find no other underlying psychiatric conditions in women who were experiencing problems. Although she is aware and understands that the objections were based upon "deeper roots" in "how this society has defined women," Severino states that she is more concerned with individual women who might have PMS.

In the same rhetorical move adopted by the Committee on Women who opposed inclusion, Severino and other proinclusion scientists made themselves into professional advocates and spokespersons for women—especially those with PMS. In Severino's mind, PMS is above all a physical or medical problem—although potentially a social problem as well. As long as women were helped, she stated that she was not as concerned about the wider implications of the diagnosis of LLPDD itself.[9]

Remarks such as these show that the issue was this: Who speaks for women? Both those favoring and opposing inclusion of LLPDD saw themselves as advancing the interests of women based upon their scientific and medical training and expertise. Both saw themselves as spokespersons for women. One major difference between the expert positions in the LLPDD debate had to do with the perceptions about the role that individual women with PMS should play in the debate. Drawing upon the time-honored position of the women's health movement, anti-inclusion experts drew upon and encouraged women with PMS to claim their own expertise about their bodies and experiences. In the next section, I focus on how individual women sought to claim their *own* voice in the debate, and how this was accomplished with empowering notions from the anti-inclusion experts and the rhetoric of feminist and women's self-help movements.

WOMEN SPEAKING FOR AND CLAIMING THEIR BODIES

The third ownership claim came from individual women who acknowledged their personal and medical history of PMS and asserted their own authority to speak for themselves as "experts" in the matter. These women with PMS (both self-diagnosed and medically diagnosed) argued that the American Psychiatric Association had no right to define "their" PMS as a psychiatric disorder. In letters of protest written to the APA, these women asserted their individually grounded expertise about PMS as a legitimate form of ownership of what they claimed was a gynecological and not a psychiatric disorder. Many women wrote multiple-paged letters to the APA describing their experiences with PMS and protesting the inclusion of LLPDD.

Support for these claims is found in the politically empowering rhetoric of the Women's Health Movement from the 1970s. The self-help movement emphasizes the explicit authority, ownership, and the right of women to control their own bodies. For example, in the popular book *The New Our Bodies, Ourselves*, The Boston Women's Health Book Collective, states: "All through this book we emphasize wherever possible what women can do—for ourselves, for each other—in staying healthy, healing ourselves and working for change" (1984a:3). They include an entire chapter on "The Politics of Women and Medical Care." Their statement about women's lack of power and control in modern health care systems suggests that

> despite our overwhelming numbers and the tremendous responsibility we carry for people's health, we have almost no power to influence the medical system. Policy makers, usually male, have designed the system primarily for the convenience and financial gain of physicians, hospitals and the medical industries. We believe that women, as the majority of consumers and work-

ers, paid and unpaid, should have the major voice in health and medical care policy-making in this country. (1984a:556)

The letters and telegrams by women have been deposited in the APA archives. They provide a wealth of data about women's attitudes toward their "illness" as something biological, not psychological or psychiatric. These women also objected strongly to the inclusion of LLPDD in DSM-III-R. The nature and themes of the letters (especially about stigmatization and gender composition of psychiatry) strongly suggest that the "campaign" orchestrated by the professional anti-inclusion forces reached individual women. These women responded to requests by the professional women to oppose the inclusion of LLPDD and to let their voices be heard by the APA leaders. Individual women also found other ways to register their voices in petitions sent from local women's centers and PMS support groups across the United States, Canada, and Great Britain, and through phone calls and telegrams directed at the APA.

There are five major themes in these women's letters.[10] First, the women asserted in various ways that they were the most qualified "experts" to speak about PMS, and in effect claimed ownership of their bodies and its by-products. In their letters to the APA, these women had a strong sense of their own authoritative voice in defining PMS as a biological and *not* as a psychiatric disorder. A woman from Kansas wrote the following in claiming her own history with PMS:

> I believe that treating women with PMS syndrome in a standard psychiatric way—disregarding the biological effects this condition has upon women—is very dangerous. It is dangerous because this condition effects many aspects of the female personality as well as her biological character. I believe that my own case history might add some insight into this problem. (undated letter)

A self-proclaimed "PMS Sufferer" in Alaska wrote:

> As a person who has suffered from PMS since puberty, I feel I know enough about the illness to write to you and let you know what a mistake it would be if this proposal [LLPDD] were to pass and PMS were to be categorized as a mental disorder. (dated June 13, 1986)

Another woman stated that

> I believe that my entire life is a testimony to the debate which the American Psychiatric Association is presently engaged in. (undated letter)

One woman from Massachusetts tried to appeal to psychiatrists' listening skills when she wrote that psychiatric training and knowledge were insufficient to really "know" about PMS:

Psychiatrists are supposed to be good listeners. I trust that you and your fellow psychiatrists will have the humility to consider the opinions of people who have much more direct experience & familiarity with the subjects at hand, and may have insights and knowledge that are beyond the scope of your experience & learning. (dated July 19, 1986)

One of the major reasons that these women did not consider their "illness" to be psychiatric was due to the biological basis and physical manifestations of their symptoms. This second theme was prevalent in most of the letters. A woman from Kansas supported the notion that because PMS is biologically based, then women can and already are being helped. She implored:

Please do not allow the American Psychiatric Association to sniff at women who have the certain knowledge that their problems have a physical basis and can be helped with medical treatment. (dated August 6, 1986)

Some women compared their PMS to other physical disorders or diseases such as diabetes:

Our condition is as simple as diabetes—cause and effect of one physical chemical imbalance is *easily* corrected. Contempt (& premature diagnosis) are signs of ignorance. You must investigate this situation more fully and be more opened [sic] minded to case histories. (dated August 25, 1986)

Epilepsy was also used as a comparison:

Calling women with PMS a mental case parallels frighteningly with labelling epileptics the same. If the same results were to occur, the APA would deserve to lose its credibility. (dated June 3, 1986)

Other women, like one from California, wrote pages of descriptions about their symptoms:

For many years I thought I was just depressed. Not all the time but enough to seem like it was all the time [my cycle is 13–15 'normal' days and 20–23 'symptomatic' days]. My symptoms are: bloating, sugar cravings, chocolate cravings, back aches, fatigue/lethargy, depression, paranoia, tension and hostility and something I can only describe as cotton in the brain. They are both physical and emotional. I have not allowed a razor blade nor a gun in my house because I was too afraid that I might use them, on myself or someone I loved. I chose not to have children because I would have killed them in a rage. (dated July 8, 1986)

An early letter written in the summer of 1985 emphasized the need for more accurate biological research on PMS:[11]

> PMS is so obviously linked to a woman's biological system that it must be categorized as a gynecological disorder if we are to get the correct kind of biological research needed to understand and treat this disorder. (dated July 24, 1985)

A woman from Texas wrote that her PMS symptoms include some psychological manifestations, but that these are insufficient to label PMS a psychiatric disorder:

> I have been diagnosed with PMS. I experience physical and psychological disorders, varying with each symptoms period. I would not be considered to have acne because I experience a zit as part of my PMS. Neither should I be considered mentally ill because I experience psychological problems with onset of PMS. (dated July, 18, 1986)

This point was echoed in a letter from a PMS support group:

> Our major concern is to help you understand and to realize that this illness definitely should not be labeled a mental disorder. It also should not be treated by psychiatric therapy alone. Having dealt with PMS personally, each one of us, for a number of years. We all know how devastating the mental symptoms of PMS can be. In the same respect we also know that no amount of counseling has helped. (dated June 9, 1986)

Other women wrote that they had no psychological or "mental" symptoms:

> I know from my personal experiences that any PMS symptoms that I may experience are not mental, and I resent the implications this revision makes that they are. (dated July 22, 1986)

Third, women wrote about the issue of labeling and stigmatization that would result if PMS were classified as psychiatric. A woman from Kansas pointed out that

> We do not call everyone mentally ill that has problems coping with an illness and I certainly fell it is very wrong to subject all the women who suffer from this into a category of a mental disorder. (undated letter)

As another woman succinctly stated:

PMS is solely a reproductive disorder. It only becomes a psychiatric problem when this sick female is given drugs or harassed. (found on an undated petition)

The concern that "new demeaning stereotypes would arise concerning all women" was the focus of a woman's letter from Minnesota:

After so many years of fighting for the respect they deserve in business, politics, and more, women will have to burden new idiotic assumptions that all their gender become violent monsters once a month, and are incapable of making decisions or taking care of themselves. (dated June 3, 1986)

Another author refused to accept the label and wondered where it would stop. She wrote:

As a longtime sufferer of PMS I object vehemently to being labeled 'mentally ill'. Or did I all at once cease to be mentally ill upon my menopause? I admit my PMS gave me some mental anguish, but so do some of my physical ails today. (dated July 15, 1986)

There were other letters from women (and one man) who did not claim to have PMS, but expressed concern over the stigmatizing effect of labeling PMS a psychiatric disorder—and its negative consequences for women. For example, a woman in Florida wrote:

My first thought after reading the proposal on PMS being a mental illness, is how is it possible to label a "mental illness" that only women experience? Why is it when a man comes home from work, snaps his wifes' [sic] head off, has no interest in sex, and just wants to be left alone—he's had a rough day at work. BUT a woman comes home with the same *exact* feelings and the consensus is that 'she's on the rag, better stay out of the way.' (dated July 1, 1986)

One woman from New York City demanded to know "why and how this could happen now. Is it a result of men being very threatened? Is it a result of trying to be 'in' with the Reagan ultra-conservatives?" (dated July 31, 1986).

These last two letters suggest an new issue related to stigmatization and make up the fourth theme: women charged that there was sexism involved in making PMS a psychiatric disorder. Some focused on the political and social aspects of the diagnostic process, and charged that the APA was basing the diagnosis upon sexist and discriminatory practices:

Many women are mindful that the psychotherapeutic sciences have not always fostered the health of women. This is an opportunity to take a healthier direction. (July 19, 1986)

In a letter to Spitzer from a woman in Texas, the notion that men cannot possibly know what women go through is explored:

> I know you as a man can not imagine what it is like to go through but you can try to understand what many women are going through. (undated letter)

Many, like the woman from Wisconsin, linked the diagnosis to the gender distribution in the psychiatric profession. She stated:

> Maybe if more than 10% of the psychiatric profession was made up of by women, the proposal to change the term never would have come up. (dated August 1, 1986)

This focus on the gender composition of the psychiatric profession was echoed by a woman in Virginia who wrote:

> When men of the medical profession start labeling PMS as a mental problem, I think it is time to start worrying! (dated July 22, 1986)

Gender composition and sexism was also the concern of a woman from New York:

> I understand that men make up 90% of the psychiatrist population. Again, as in the anti-abortion issues, men are making rules and issuing rulings for women which involve issues outside of their personal experience. (dated July 12, 1986)

This same woman added the fifth theme, the charge of economic motivation and interests of the APA. She concluded her letter by saying:

> I realize that the new labeling would cultivate for psychiatrists a new area for getting insurance reimbursements given only for diseases sanctioned by the Diagnostic and Statistical Manual. (dated July 12, 1986)

From California, a woman wrote of economic interests as well as sexism. She wrote:

> Categories such as those proposed continue to portray women as victims and create further avenues of revenue for the overwhelmingly male psychiatric profession from insurance companies. SO DROP THEM! (dated July 22, 1986)

This sentiment was joined by a woman from Pennsylvania:

This will only lead to degrading women. It will also just line the pockets of the psychiatrists unnecessarily. Then, too, the psychiatrists (especially the 90% who are male) have never understood or even tried to understand Pre-Menstrual Syndrome. Perhaps it is because the great majority of psychiatrists have entered the field of psychiatry because they need mental help themselves. (dated July 12, 1986)

"Why is this being done?" asked a woman from Pennsylvania. Her answer:

I suspect economic reasons—not a medical one. No doubt someone stands to make more dollars from insurance if the name is changed. And as usual, women are being labelled to benefit a power structure run (mainly) by white males. (dated July 21, 1986).

There are no examples of what might be considered a proinclusion letter from any individual woman.[12] Most nonprofessional women who wrote a letter or signed a petition strongly believed that PMS exists biologically and that its inclusion as a psychiatric diagnosis would be harmful to this "fact" and to women's interests.

In spite of making their views and presence known during the debate, why weren't these women with PMS the main focus of controversy over the inclusion of LPPDD in the DSM-III-R? Why were the individual women's voices who have PMS usually ignored in the controversy? Part of the answer lies in the way that the DSM is revised within the organizational structure of the APA (see Chapter 3 for a complete review of this process).

Bell's 1987 analysis of the medicalization of PMS suggested something called "points of contest" among professionals interested in PMS.[13] She focuses upon what she calls "arenas of contest" within the larger process of medicalization. She states that "[t]he process of medicalization is complex, and the stages are contained in a number of different arenas of contest. First, there are intraprofessional and interprofessional disputes over the etiology and treatment of PMS. In addition to controversy within and between gynecology and psychiatry, there is controversy in psychology and the law" (Bell 1987:156).

Bell's point is significant. The controversy over psychiatric manifestations of PMS was not in the hands of the individual women who experience it every month. Rather, it moved under the control of experts in many forms: health or mental health professions (in Chapter 5), scientists and researchers (in Chapter 7), or even professional women in these occupations or professional advocates of the feminist and women's health movements.

The individual women with PMS—concerned about the possible stigmatization of LLPDD—expressed themselves in the only means available to them: through letters, telegrams, or phone calls. They asserted their individually grounded expertise with PMS as a legitimate form of ownership of what they claimed was a biological (not psychiatric) disorder. These moves empowered the powerless person to feel like at least they had tried to make their own voices heard in the sea of professional and medical "expert" voices.

THE GENDERED NATURE OF THE CONTROVERSY

Together in the woman domain of analysis, these three ownership claims (those made for women with PMS and those made by women with PMS) constituted and constructed LLPDD as a gendered issue. As such, the ownership claims in this domain are situated within the context of research and arguments made in the feminist and women's health literatures. How the claims were expressed differed according to the structural position of participants, and is then related to ownership claims over LLPDD.

Whereas professional advocates were claiming to speak on behalf of all women, women with self- or professionally diagnosed cases of PMS were demanding that they could also speak for themselves. Women's health and feminist organizations argued that psychiatric labeling of PMS and LLPDD by the American Psychiatric Association was not scientifically based and also harmful to all women. Proinclusion scientists argued that the diagnosis of LLPDD would legitimate the psychological symptoms of PMS as something real and not just in women's heads. The third ownership claim was made by women with PMS (both self-diagnosed and medically diagnosed) that the American Psychiatric Association had no authority to define PMS as a psychiatric disorder.

These three ownership claims constituted and constructed LLPDD as a woman's issue—centered on the basic issue of medicalization of women's bodies and the stigmatization of a gender-specific mental illness. Although by no means "determining" the rhetoric and arguments of the gendered ownership claims, feminist literature formed and informed the participant's rhetorical and political positions in the debate. For example, the connection of a psychiatric diagnosis with women's menstrual cycles—and its potential applicability to all women—was expressed as the major concern by individuals and in statements from women's and feminist organizations. Whereas professional advocates were speaking as "experts" on behalf of all women, their rhetoric, knowledge, arguments, and even their "selves" were situated within the feminist and women's health literature. The individual women with PMS also drew upon the feminist and women's health literature by demanding that they could speak for themselves, with their own knowledge about their bodies and health experiences.

There are positive consequences of calling peoples' attention to the gendered and therefore political nature of this diagnosis. The controversy was indeed recognized as a "woman's" or "feminist" issue. Public attention was focused upon the gender politics involved in the creation of medical and psychiatric diagnoses. More people became aware that even science and medicine are political and gendered.

The Committee on Women of the APA engaged in a successful coalition-building and tactical campaign that resulted in the placement of the diagnosis in a research appendix of DSM-III-R. The alternative would have been the inclusion of a diagnosis called Premenstrual Dysphoric Disorder in the main text. The inclusion of Late Luteal Phase Dysphoric Disorder in the appendix ensured that more systematic and standardized scientific research—needed to justify or delete its existence in the next manual—would be undertaken.

But there were personal costs for members of the Committee on Women. In the end, Bernardez stated that she and others who fought the inclusion of LLPDD felt that they had to "pull away" and "abandon" the American Psychiatric Association. She stated that up until the point of the DSM-III-R controversy, there was hope and change in the APA for women and feminist perspectives: "They destroyed all possible hopes of change in psychiatry" (personal interview, April 20, 1990, East Lansing). This sentiment of personal loss and hurt was echoed by Hamilton who stated that "I feel like a battered woman. I feel like I was emotionally battered in trying to pursue this area of work [by being at the center of the controversy]. I would not do it over again" (personal interview, June 4, 1990, Washington, D.C.).

Another negative consequence of making LLPDD a public issue occurred as a result of the way in which professional expertise and advocacy of the feminist and women's health experts were diminished in both the public and scientific/medical presses. This was accomplished was by a blanket labeling of all opposition to inclusion of the diagnosis as "feminist" (i.e., the "Political Account"). Even in the early accounts of the controversy in the American Psychological Association's bulletin, *The APA Monitor*, the issue was portrayed as a battle between feminists and psychiatrists (although the anti-inclusion people quoted in the article were all members of the psychological association). "Three proposed new categories—masochistic personality disorder, paraphilic rapism and premenstrual dysphoric disorder,—have been amended slightly after feminist critics called the original language 'anti-female'" (Fisher 1986a:17).[14] An account in *The Washington Post* put all opposition under the label of "feminist":

> The nation's leading psychiatric organization has proposed labeling premenstrual syndrome a mental illness, triggering protests from feminists who

fear such a move will stigmatize women professionally and personally. (DePaul 1986:20)

This public portrayal of the protest as merely "feminist" or "political" has not been lost on those labeled "feminists." In a published commentary "Is Media Coverage on the Diagnostic Controversy an Index of History in-the-making for Women in Science?," Jean Hamilton makes the argument that "The 'feminist' label in particular, is often sufficient to strip the individual of the role of 'scientist'; and to confer marginal, pseudo-scientific status, or even downright invisibility as a scientist" (1987/1988:9). The irony is that in their role of speaking for all women and claiming for women the right to define and control their bodies, these women psychiatrists, scientists, psychologists, and social workers were made to lose their credentials as "legitimate" scholars and practitioners. They became the ubiquitous "feminist" protester—scientifically and professionally defrocked.

Inclusion of LLPDD in the DSM-III-R even in the appendix (and especially with a psychiatric coding) signaled a defeat for professional women who fought its inclusion anywhere and for women who now could be labeled "having a mental illness." As feminist analyst Jacquelyn Zita commented:

> It is no accident that a culture threatened by the erasure of gender differences as criteria for discrimination and domination would try to reinstate the social significance of such differences though its most legitimate authority— science. (Zita 1988:94)

The issue of how and why the authority and legitimacy of science settled the issue of LLPDD is explored in the next chapter.

NOTES

1. See Clarke (1990a:15) for a recent analysis of the impact and criticisms of Ehrenreich and English's work.

2. See Loring and Powell (1988) for a description and analysis of this study.

3. One need only point to the origin for the word hysteria, which was derived from the Greek word "hystera," which means uterus.

4. Information located in the personal archives of Dr. Jean Hamilton at the Institute for Research on Women's Health in Washington, D.C. and the Archives of the American Psychiatric Association, Washington, D.C.

5. Letter found in the personal archives of Dr. Jean Hamilton at the Institute for Research on Women's Health, Washington, D.C.

6. Letter found in the personal archives of Dr. Jean Hamilton at the Institute for Research on Women's Health, Washington, D.C..

7.   According to Hamilton, the most active people at the Institute of Research on Women's Health in terms of spending time fighting the diagnosis were herself, psychologist and co-author Sheryl Gallant, social worker Linda King, and psychologist Jackie Gentry: "Those were the people who actually sat here and helped stuff envelopes and put on stamps and all on this stuff" (Hamilton, personal interview, June 4, 1990, Washington, D.C.).

8.   This booklet was prepared by Dr. Hamilton and her colleagues for the National Coalition for Women's Mental Health and formed the basis of Hamilton's presentation about LLPDD at the APA's Annual Meeting in May 1986.

9.   These data are based upon a personal interview with Dr. Severino, which took place on May 24, 1991 in White Plains, New York.

10.   I have not included the names or any personal identifying features of these women. Their letters are located in the Archives of the American Psychiatric Association in Washington, D.C. This decision was not done to further ignore their voice but rather to listen in a way that focuses upon the arguments and feelings that they express.

11.   A note accompanying the copy of this particular letter indicates that copies were sent to Dr. Spitzer and to Dr. Carol Nadelson, then President of the APA.

12.   This fact is probably due to the success of the forces that mobilized against the diagnosis and not because some women did not support the idea the PMS could be a psychiatric disorder.

13.   This paper was written during the early stages of the LLPDD controversy. Bell's paper stemmed from a 1984 conference and was not published until 1987. She does not specifically address the DSM-III-R issues but focuses upon the ways in which the then proposed diagnosis of "Premenstrual Dysphoric Disorder" was yet another example of the institutionalization of PMS.

14.   However, by the next story about the controversy in the APA Monitor, the ubiquitous term "feminist" was replaced with the phrase "feminist psychologists and psychiatrists and others" (see Fisher July 1986a:4).

7

The "Truth" about PMS and LLPDD:
The Science Domain

Science, since people must do it, is a socially embedded activity. It progresses by hunch, vision, and intuition. Much of its change through time does not
record a closer approach to absolute truth, but the alteration of cultural contexts that influence it so strongly. Facts are not pure and unsullied bits of information; culture also influences what we see and how we see it. (Gould
1981:21–22)

In the "Science Domain," LLPDD is an occasion for contesting the control
and ownership of the "scientific truth" or "reality" about PMS. Throughout the controversy over inclusion of LLPDD in DSM-III-R, the debate focused upon the scientific validity of claims about PMS and on the research
implications of creating LLPDD as a psychiatric diagnosis. Debate over the
scientific validity of LLPDD focuses attention on the nature and settlement
of controversy in science and medicine. Identifying the array of people, interests, discourses, and events that were pivotal in defining LLPDD as an
artifact of science and of scientists is essential for mapping out the science
domain. This is achieved in several ways.

The boundaries of the science domain are first set by reviewing contemporary literature in the sociology of science and technology. As with
the other two domains, the sociological literature is reviewed not just to
show its relevance for understanding the preconstituted entity called
LLPDD. Rather, in the science domain, the sociology of science (alongside
participants and their discourse) constitutes LLPDD—gives it definition,
shape, and meaning—as an object of scientific fact and truth about the psychological manifestations of PMS. As the introductory quotation from
Stephen J. Gould suggests, science is a social activity and the knowledge
produced by scientists is embedded within cultural notions, political interests, and societal goals.

This domain of analysis is also constructed by looking at historical and contemporary scientific and medical debates about PMS and LLPDD. Debates among scientists about the truth and validity of PMS and LLPDD were important factors in explaining why the LLPDD controversy proceeded as it did in the scientific community. In the end, "science" and scientific authority temporarily settled the issue of LLPDD. How and why LLPDD became a legitimate scientific artifact are explored by situating the debate in a literature that draws attention to other, similar scientific controversies.

THE SOCIOLOGY OF SCIENTIFIC KNOWLEDGE

The sociology of scientific knowledge (SSK) perspective does not emphasize the study of the institution of science nor the careers of scientists (Knorr-Cetina 1983; Bijker, Hughes and Pinch 1987; Woolgar 1988). Instead, drawing on developments in the history and philosophy of science (i.e., Kuhn's [(1962) 1970] work on scientific revolutions), the SSK focus is on the construction of scientific knowledge in society. Woolgar summarizes the constructivist perspective:

> the sociologist could no longer accept as given the distinction between true and false scientific beliefs. Instead, the sociological task was to discern what counts as true and false belief; in particular, what social processes are involved in the construction, assessment and evaluation of knowledge. (Woolgar 1988:41)

Constructivist studies have shifted analytic attention away from the social institution of science to the content of knowledge created by scientists. As early as 1935, Fleck argued that scientific facts are not "discovered" but "invented." Constructivists would not assume that LLPDD is a mirror of reality, or that women "really" experience their bodies in this way. By contrast, realists assume that scientific truths mirror nature, and that nature adjudicates among knowledge-claims—selecting for "truth" those that correspond to external reality.

In SSK, the existence of LLPDD is a knowledge-claim constructed by scientists for identifiable reasons. Those "reasons" are labeled "interests" by the Edinburgh school of constructivism (Barnes 1977; Mackenzie 1981; Bloor 1981). Something other than nature shapes the social construction of scientific facts. For example, Pickering uses an "opportunism-in-context" model to understand how the particle physics community "constructed" quarks. The founding of high-energy physics (or LLPDD and psychiatric studies of PMS, for that matter) "can be understood in terms of the particular resources and context of the individuals concerned, just as the elaboration of those traditions can be understood in terms of the shared resources and contexts of the groups involved" (Pickering 1984:13). Pickering and other interest sociologists would ask: Why were some scientists interested in the creation of LLPDD and not others? How would some scientists gain—and others lose—if LLPDD were to become real?

The interest model also demonstrates a congruence between a person's social position and their courses of action (Mackenzie 1981). Scientists occupy different social positions and from these, they try to maximize various material and social resources. Thus, interests constrain (not determine) beliefs and actions appropriate to the social positions. For example, biopsychiatrists interested in mood or hormonal disorders might be more interested in the creation of the scientific artifact of LLPDD than would social workers or psychologists who take a behavioral approach to mental disorders. As Law states:

> Because social groups have different interests and resources, they tend to have different views of the proper structure of artifacts. Accordingly, the stabilization of artifacts is explained by referring to social interests that are imputed to the groups concerned and their differential capacity to mobilize resources in the course of debate and controversy. (Law 1987:111)

To summarize, from the "Edinburgh" perspective, the reality (or fiction) of LLPDD becomes a vehicle for some scientists to advance their material or symbolic interests.

Constructivist studies have also empirically displayed the socially situated, contextually contingent, and constructed nature of scientific knowledge in a wide variety of disciplines, sites, and periods (Latour and Woolgar 1979; Pickering 1984; Shapin 1984). Public and private discourse of scientists has become a valuable source of information about how facts are socially constructed. SSK has also shown how the profession of science has been more successful than other forms of knowledge in getting people to believe in the efficacy and truth of its explanations of the world (Gieryn 1983; Latour 1987, 1988). This line of inquiry opens up for study the mechanisms through which scientists persuade other actors such as business leaders, politicians, and the press to accept their beliefs and support their work. This focus has provided an important sociological explanation (i.e., empirically grounded, rather than philosophical) for the growth of scientific knowledge, authority, and expertise.

Recently, SSK has expanded its range by incorporating a "systems" or network approach to the study of science and technology. The Social Construction of Technology (SCOT) has extended SSK's focus on facts to include the social construction of artifacts (see the articles in Pinch and Bijker 1987). How, why, and in whose interests did certain kinds of technological artifacts develop and others not? This perspective allows researchers to analyze how the technical (or scientific) aspects of an artifact are connected with its social and political aspects.

The main point of SCOT studies is that the technical is social. In Langdon Winner's terms, artifacts have politics, and it is the job of the analyst to identify connections between the two (1980). This orientation simultaneously makes LLPDD into scientific knowledge (fact) and a technology (artifact). Analytically, there is no difference between the two; facts are made, just like machines. One could argue that LLPDD is not "technically" a technological artifact in the sense of a product bought and sold in a commercial market. Or is it? The SCOT perspective suggests that LLPDD gets used as research and diagnostic criteria or tool in grant proposals, articles, or studies. LLPDD is not just the knowledge but the tools (or technology) used to study PMS. For this reasons, LLPDD is copyrighted by the American Psychiatric Association as part of a larger research and diagnostic tool, the DSM-III-R. It thus becomes an artifact bought and sold in the medical, mental health, and scientific marketplace. As a product or tool of science, the APA does not widely advertise the DSM-III-R, but it certainly does in relevant scientific or medical journals.

In summary, LLPDD becomes many things when constituted by SSK. It is something manufactured by scientists into "fact." Different scientists have various interests in the reality of PMS, and the existence of LLPDD is shaped by these interests. Finally, LLPDD is a technology with politics. It is an artifact bought and sold in a market. The goal of the SSK analyst is to show the connections between the technical character of LLPDD and the social processes that go into its making. According to SSK, LLPDD becomes a socially constructed scientific and technical artifact. But no privilege, authority, or objectivity is attached to *this* sociological account. As SSK helps remind us, one account is analytically equivalent to other stories, and another account of LLPDD is presented in the next section.

SCIENTIFIC AND TECHNICAL CONTROVERSIES

Newspapers, television, popular magazines, and scientific journals all carry news about controversies related to science and technology. Scientific and technical controversies are an important area of study for sociologists, with a long and rich history (Nelkin 1982, 1992; Peterson and Markle 1980; McCrea 1983; Martin 1991).

Sociologists have shown that controversies in science or medicine have important social, economic, and political consequences—not only for society-at-large but for scientific-medical communities as well. Sociologists of science have studied public issues ranging from the building of airports (Nelkin 1992) to the use of fluoridation in the water system (Martin 1991) to the role of scientists in the acid rain debate (Zehr 1990). Controversy studies raise questions about the role of scientists and scientific knowledge in settling public issues with scientific or technical dimensions. How do scientists maintain their public authority—based in larger measure of assumptions of rationality—in these partisan controversies?

When constituted by this sociological literature, LLPDD becomes another scientific and technical controversy. It was first a controversy among experts (scientists, psychiatrists, psychologists, and gynecologists) debating the "truth" of PMS. It then became a public issue for discussion among women, feminists, and women's organizations who entered the debate with their own "experts." Who would the public believe about LLPDD? Not only were scientific experts disagreeing among themselves about PMS, but private citizens and political organizations became actively involved. How do scientists on both sides of an issue use—and preserve—the authority of science when scientific controversies enter the realm of political debate?

These controversies often get settled through a rhetorical exploitation of the authority of science, brought in to bolster arguments (see Gieryn and Figert 1986, 1990). When scientific controversies go public and when scientific experts offer discrepant versions of reality as "truth," the authority of science itself is at risk. Because scientists and other professionals claim to have the "truth" and "the facts" by virtue of their training and education, public disputes among professionals could hurt their professional credibility and standing. If "truth" and "facts" are contested among doctors and scientists, who then is the public to believe? Is PMS a psychiatric disorder, a gynecological disorder, or not a disorder at all? If LLPDD was built using "faulty" data and methodologies, what is the right way to study PMS? Who decides and settles scientific controversies?

Assumptions about the rational nature of scientific discourse and methodology are important factors in how scientific controversies get settled. As Dorothy Nelkin points out:

> The authority of scientific expertise has rested on assumptions about scientific rationality. The interpretations and predictions of scientists are judged to be rational and immune to political manipulation because they are based on data gathered through objective procedures. (1992:xviii)

In addition, when scientific debates become public, they begin to take on an even more esoteric "technical" nature. For example, Gilbert and Mulkay (1984) find that scientists use an entirely different form of discourse when talking in public, as opposed to when they talk among themselves informally in laboratories or at conferences. In employing these "empiricist repertoires" on public occasions, scientists present information in a way that preempts debate about its legitimacy. Gilbert and Mulkay state:

Each scientist's actions and beliefs, no matter how inconsistent they appear to be with those of other researchers, are presented as those of any competent scientist. The guiding principle of this repertoire appears to be that speakers depict their actions and beliefs as a neutral medium through with empirical phenomena make themselves evident. (1984:56)

Validity rests with "nature," not with its representation.

Social, economic, and political values become difficult to distinguish from scientific facts during scientific and technical controversies. Power employed by different actors in settling scientific disputes "hinges on the ability to manipulate knowledge, to challenge the evidence presented to support particular policies, and technical expertise becomes a resource exploited by all parties to justify their political and economic views" (Nelkin 1979:17). This is important for understanding the settlement of the LLPDD controversy.

LLPDD AS CONSTRUCTED BY SOCIOLOGY OF SCIENCE LITERATURES

In the science domain, perspectives from constructivist studies of science and sociological studies of scientific and technical controversies constitute LLPDD as a scientific artifact. How? Each points to the social, political, and economic nature of scientific practices, and to the publicly negotiated and constructed nature of scientific facts and knowledge. LLPDD becomes a scientific artifact, but with none of the positivist or realist assumptions typically attached to "science." It is a socially constructed cultural artifact whose existence owes less to nature than to the political and economic interests its reality would serve.

LLPDD is not a mirror of reality per se but a measure of scientists' pragmatic interests and debate in this public and private controversy. As Star recently pointed out, constructivists share certain assumptions: "Among our common interests and beliefs was the necessity of 'opening up the black box' in order to demystify science and technology, that is, to analyze the process of production as well as the product. The methodological directives here for us were familiar: understand the language and meanings of your respondents, link them with institutional patterns and commitments, and as Everett Hughes said 'it could have been otherwise'" (as quoted in Star 1988:198).

The preceding discussion had lead up to the discussion of another account of LLPDD—as a scientific artifact. This account was done by PMS scientists, researchers, and actors also involved in the LLPDD controversy.

These accounts provide yet another interpretive context in which LLPDD settled in the appendix of DSM-III-R.

THE SCIENCE OF PMS AND ITS RESEARCHERS

What scientifically constitutes PMS—and how PMS research should be legitimately carried out—were questions raised from within science and from outside, political critics. These questions shaped both the debate and settlement of LLPDD as a scientific artifact. The aim (and possibly its result as well) of feminist scientific work on menstruation was to refute negative images of PMS using the tools and rhetoric of science. Change in public perception and attitudes about the previously understudied topic of menstruation and PMS was thought to be achievable from within the halls of science.

The nature and content of pre-1980s PMS research—and those who carried it out—are important parts of the developing story of LLPDD. In 1983, Abplanalp characterized PMS research in the following manner: because PMS symptoms are behavioral, psychological, and physiological in nature, "researchers from the biological as well as the social sciences have contributed to the PMS research literature" (Abplanalp 1983:107). All types of scientific research (social science as well as biological science) were being conducted and funded by different types of researchers (biologists, gynecologists, psychologists, and psychiatrists).

But, according to Koeske, the major difference among PMS researchers was whether they held a purely biological/biomedical orientation or a feminist and thus more sociocultural orientation (1983). As discussed in Chapter 6, a feminist or sociocultural perspective challenges traditional bio-medical control of women's bodies and experiences. A bio-medical orientation to PMS considers it a medical problem requiring specific types of scientific research, diagnosis, and intervention (Parlee 1992). These differences among PMS researchers played an important role in shaping PMS and in the development of LLPDD.

THE 1983 CONFERENCE AND SCIENTIFICALLY DEFINING PMS

A marked shift in the PMS research community took place at a May 1983 conference sponsored by the National Institute of Mental Health (NIMH). This conference played a major role in bringing together a diverse group of research scientists, psychiatrists, and psychologists who were then doing PMS-related research. The main product of this 1983 NIMH conference was a working scientific definition of Premenstrual Syndrome: "a diagnosis of premenstrual syndrome should be made when symptom intensity changes at least 30% in the premenstrual period (6 days before menses) compared with the intermenstrual period (days 5–10 of the cycle) for two consecutive months" (Blume 1983; Osofsky and Blumenthal 1985:88).

The 1983 definition of PMS was seen as a scientific advance in a field in which no previous agreement or definition had been reached. A consistent definition could tighten research and clinical standards of evaluation. This was important for a researcher at the conference whose grant proposal had been rejected with the following comment: "You want to study something that does not exist with methods that are inadequate" (as reported in Blume 1983:2866). According to Jean Hamilton: "The concern was basically, look, NIMH isn't currently funding anything and they are not going to do it unless it's a diagnosis" (personal interview, June 4, 1990). This sentiment was echoed during the LLPDD debate by another PMS researcher:

> The few clinical scientists with the interest and wherewithal to make a concerted effort to address many of the unresolved issues about premenstrual syndrome are faced, on one hand, with the concern that their peers will not accord their research proposals sufficient priority to ensure funding at times of government cutbacks and, on the other hand, with the fear that editors of first-rate scientific journals may ultimately refuse to publish the results of research on premenstrual syndrome for fear that this quasiscientific 'quality of life' issue might not conform to the rigid scientific standards expected by their readership. (Reid 1986:923)

The 1983 NIMH conference did not fully resolve all definitional and methodological issues of PMS research. Scientists (on both sides of the LLPDD debate) still pointed to the lack of clarity and to the absence of solid scientific data to fully support it as a diagnosis (see Hamilton and Alagna 1988; Severino and Moline 1989). More research was called for, given the increasing level of interest in PMS by the public and by other health and mental health professionals.

Public interest in scientific research is generally perceived by researchers as vital. In fact, Johnson points out that the impetus and pressure for PMS research came not from within the scientific community but from consumers or the public. He states: "it has primarily been pressure from the lay public which has resulted in movement within the medical profession to specifically address PMS" (Johnson 1987:341). A "proper" public image of PMS research was important for reasons both external and internal to the scientific community. If PMS research was seen as inconclusive and plagued by methodological or epistemological difficulties, it might not get funded by government agencies and other patrons, or published by scientific journals. If some scientists do not perceive PMS research as legitimate science, then the public might not believe PMS experts or seek out their advice and treatments.

According to scientific and medical reports of the 1983 NIMH conference in the *Journal of the American Medical Association* (JAMA), panelists "were hard-pressed to define the disorder precisely and seemed all too aware that their research is plagued with methodological difficulties" (Blume 1983:2866). Even well-known and respected PMS researchers noted in the *American Journal of Psychiatry* that "despite 50 years of study, no commonly agreed-on definition of premenstrual syndrome exists, no biochemical correlates have been systematically identified, and no treatment has been consistently demonstrated to be more effective than placebo in well-designed double-bind studies" (Rubinow et al., 1984:684). In an editorial in the *New England Journal of Medicine*, another PMS researcher pointed out that "[v]ery little is understood about the patho-physiology of the syndrome, and there is much speculation" (Vaitukaitis 1984:1372). Representations of problems in PMS research that appeared in the scientific press did not pose as big a problem for the scientists' authority and credibility as when they went "public" and became lay knowledge.

Reports about methodological difficulties of scientific and medical research on PMS were indeed making their way into the popular press. A *Vogue* reprint of a 1984 *Harvard Medical School Health Letter*, printed at the same time that the LLPDD Advisory Committee was meeting to decide to include PDD in DSM-III-R, informed its readers that:

> The symptoms of PMS are hard enough to pin down, and effective therapies are even more in dispute. One reason for this difficulty is that the evidence underlying most of the popular treatments is suggestive rather than scientific. . . . The few PMS studies that have been properly controlled to avoid distorted observation have generally been too small and too brief to be conclusive. (1985:306)

An article in *Ms.* magazine informed its readers that: "While PMS is now generally acknowledged to be a physical, as well as a psychological disorder, there is little agreement on what causes it or how it should be treated. There are at least half a dozen theories as to its cause—ranging from an alteration in the way that the body uses glucose, to excessive estrogen levels—none of which have been convincingly demonstrated" (Eagan 1983:28).

This perception of scientific uncertainty conveyed by the public press was not necessarily a bad thing for scientists and PMS researchers. Because PMS was portrayed as the "new" disease of the 1980s, uncertainty meant that funding and more research were needed. Science and medicine had not, yet, come up with "answers" about PMS. But with proper support and attention from scientists and health professionals, science would eventually provide them. PMS researcher/gynecologist Reid reports:

> Increased public awareness about premenstrual syndrome and a growing sense of personal responsibility for wellness among health care consumers are bringing unprecedented numbers of women to our offices in search of solutions for adverse premenstrual experiences, which, a mere decade ago, were accepted as an inevitable part of being female. Whether we personally view premenstrual syndrome as fad, fact, or fallacy, it is timely for each of us to reexamine not only our own attitudes and biases but also the external influences that may have directed our thinking on this issue. (Reid 1986:921)

Scientific, medical, and popular reports of scientific and methodological difficulties in defining and studying PMS did play an important role in the development of LLPDD. Those favoring inclusion of LLPDD argued that the methodological and scientific standards of PMS research would be raised and codified.[1] At first, from the standpoint of LLPDD opposition leader Hamilton, "it was quite surprising, at least from a scientific viewpoint, that only several years later that people were trying to make a diagnosis based on what they said before was poor data" (personal interview, Hamilton, June 4, 1990, Washington, D.C.).

But the decision to include a PMS-related diagnosis was not surprising to others familiar with trends toward biopsychological analysis and treatment. According to an article written before the initial creation of LLPDD, "[t]he rise of PMS can be traced to recent trends in psychiatry, especially a closer union with neurology and its search for biochemical factors in any mental disorder. PMS was a prime candidate for this new approach" (Heneson 1984:67).

Evidence for a link between trends in psychiatry, the definition of PMS created at the 1983 NIMH conference, and subsequent development of LLPDD is found in many accounts. Jean Hamilton was a participant at the 1983 NIMH conference. In her view, this meeting was the source of the idea of getting a premenstrual diagnosis into the DSM-III-R. She states that:

> [I]t was at that meeting that I became concerned that there was a move afoot to create a psychiatric diagnosis related to PMS and I think many people saw that forewarning as sort of coming out of the blue. But the people who had been invited were the people like Jean Endicott who were very much into making diagnoses. I mean, that's sort of their bread and butter. That's their trade. And so I could see it coming. (personal interview, Hamilton, June 4,1990)

According to Spitzer, consideration of PMS came out of his interest in what constitutes a mental disorder. But, he acknowledges that the National Institute of Mental Health did play a role. He stated:

> So having given a lot of thought to what is a mental disorder, in my own mind I had clearly decided that ideology was of no issue. So it was of no concern to me whether PMS had or did not have some kind of biological affinity. The issue for me just was, was it really an independent . . . did it have some validity as an independent behavioral syndrome. . . . So with that thought I then touched base with people at NIMH . . . and we arranged that first meeting [in June 1985] and that's how it started. (personal interview, May 23, 1991)

In their clinical guide to PMS research, Severino and Moline state that interest in PMS among mental health professionals was a positive force because it led to the creation of LLPDD:

> The [1983] NIMH conference itself reflected the increasing interest of mental health professionals in PMS. The reason that premenstrual syndrome has attracted such attention in the mental health field is because of the prominence of mood disturbance in most women who have menstrually related symptoms sufficiently severe to cause them to seek clinical attention. (Severino and Moline 1989:20)

The connection is further discussed in an article written by an NIMH official and a former APA president:

> The work of the [1983] NIMH group was furthered by the establishment of a committee in 1985 to develop a diagnostic category for premenstrual syndrome to be included in the DSM-III-R. The purpose of developing such a category was to establish a set of rigorous operational criteria for definitional purposes to achieve comparability of research findings across studies and to facilitate communication among health care professionals and their patients and between researchers and clinicians. (Gitlin and Pasnau 1989:470)

These quotations provide a direct link between movements in biopsychiatry, the NIMH conference, and the creation of LLPDD.

Scientists' response to scientific and public accounts of PMS was important for other reasons. Given the confused slate of symptoms and treatment possibilities, PMS attracted many "alternative" healers with "nonscientific" treatments and prescriptions. If PMS was indeed the "disease of the 1980s" then scientists needed to ensure that its study was "legitimate science," clearly demarcated from "quackery" or scientifically "unsound" treatments. For example, one article discussing PMS research and researchers noted:

Rubinow, like many other serious scientists, is aware that lengthy research projects can leave suffering victims without much recourse for the time being. They worry that progesterone, heavily promoted by commercial PMS clinics, may become the 1980s equivalent of Lydia Pinkham's Vegetable Compound, the 19th-century remedy for 'female complaint' whose chief active ingredient was alcohol. (Heneson 1984:71)

One way to ensure scientist's control of PMS was to codify its definition and formally outline "legitimate" treatment protocols.

The definition of PMS and further delineations of LLPDD were two ways that "boundary-work" between science and nonscience occurred (Gieryn 1983). Boundary-work is defined as "the attribution of selected characteristics to the institution of science (i.e., to its practitioners, methods, stock of knowledge, values and work organization) for purposes of constructing a social boundary that distinguishes some intellectual activities as non-science" (Gieryn 1983:782). Creating definitions and diagnoses served the interests of the scientific community in preserving PMS and LLPDD as areas of "scientific" research and practice. Traditional healers were excluded and thus denied the cultural authority typically associated with science.

The 1983 NIMH conference and later interpretations of its guidelines played an important role in the controversy over LLPDD. The apparent lack of scientific consensus about symptoms and treatments of PMS was played out by scientists in two different ways: First, beginning with the strategy supported by proinclusion researchers, efforts were made to push for a PMS-related psychiatric diagnosis in the revision of the DSM-III. Second, inclusion would ensure its scientific legitimation as a psychiatric disorder and was needed to secure funding for further scientific/medical research.

THE SCIENTIFIC DEBATE ABOUT PMS AND LLPDD

With the adoption of LLPDD, the psychiatric community could be seen as responding positively to a felt "need" in the society-at-large to address the problems of women with PMS. According to proinclusion scientist Barbara Parry in the 1986 APA Annual Meeting debate:

Now, more than ever, we need diagnostic criteria for PMDD [LLPDD] to curb the abuse of this diagnosis and to foster clinical and scientific research. (as quoted in the *News Bulletin of the American Psychiatric Association* 1986)

According to other proinclusion scientists, the classification of PMS in the DSM-III-R "confers legitimacy on a syndrome historically neglected by doctors and scientists" (as quoted in De Paul 1986:20). David Rubinow, a member of the LLPDD committee and PMS researcher, stated that in spite of feminists' concerns "this is a gain for feminists" (as quoted in Holden 1986:231). He further asserted professional expertise: "It's a mental disorder. . . . Anyone who doesn't believe that hasn't worked with these people (PMS sufferers)" (as quoted in DePaul 1986:20).

Sally Severino was the other proinclusion scientist involved in the debate at the APA convention. She argued that LLPDD is a much more focused and delineated diagnosis. "Women label themselves as having PMDD [LLPDD] . . . so why stigmatize them further by not allowing them a diagnosis" (as quoted in the *News Bulletin of the American Psychiatric Association* 1986). Because LLPDD was narrowly defined to include only those women who had severe psychological manifestations, proinclusion supporters claimed that it would allow for distinctions among women who have PMS symptoms. As Rubinow succinctly stated: the inclusion of the diagnosis "will make it clear that the great majority of women do not suffer from 'raging hormones'" (Holden 1986:231).

The second reaction, held by anti-inclusion researchers, argued that more research was needed and that not enough conclusive scientific data existed to support the inclusion of what became LLPDD in DSM-III-R. As presented in documents that opponents of LLPDD faxed and mailed all over the world: "The scientific data have not proven that the 'Menstrual Cycle' causes any specific syndrome."[2] At the APA debate in May 1986 an anti-inclusion handout made available to all in attendance also emphasized in capitalized and bold letters that "RESEARCH EVIDENCE DOES NOT SUPPORT THE PMDD DIAGNOSIS (PREMENSTRUAL DYSPHORIC DISORDER)."

Jean Hamilton and Sheryl Alagna presented the anti-inclusion arguments. Two main "scientific" points were presented as evidence for not including a PMS-related diagnosis in the DSM-III-R.[3] First, correlation does not mean causation. Hamilton and Alagna's point was that the LLPDD diagnosis confused the correlation of dysphoria (bad moods) and the premenstrual phase with its cause. Second, Hamilton and Alagna argued that PMS data are primarily based upon self-report studies. Knowledge of participating in a menstrually related study elevates "negative affect/dysphoria self-ratings by about 28–76 percent." If women know that they are participating in a PMS study, they are more likely to notice negative symptoms and to report them. Double-blind studies that obscure participant's self-reports are needed.[4]

Hamilton and Alagna explicitly argued that political "boundary-work" was the main focus of the debate, instead of scientific discussion: "[O]ur opposition to the diagnosis is not simply or even primarily political; our opposition is first and foremost as scientists and our concern is with the lack of scientific evidence for the diagnosis."[5] Remember that identifica-

tion of opposition scientists as "feminists" served to make the public discussion of the artifact a purely political matter (see Hamilton 1988). In the
August edition of the *Psychiatric Times* report of the Board of Trustees meeting in which LLPDD was placed in an appendix comes the statement:

> Several observers expressed dismay at the Board's actions. A concern stated
> was that the Board of Trustees has capitulated to feminist political pressures,
> turning its back on hard scientific evidence. (August 1986)

For many, the LLPDD controversy was entirely about "feminist" politics,
and not at all about the "scientific truth" of PMS or about the sufficiency
of "scientific" evidence warranting inclusion of LLPDD in the DSM-III-R.
In spite of the many scientific arguments made by anti-inclusion actors,
their opposition was often portrayed as thoroughly "political" and not
"scientific." As Hamilton told me:

> Part of the irony is that the proponents of the diagnosis were making politi-
> cal arguments and yet they characterized us as being these anonymous fem-
> inists, who clearly couldn't have a scientific thought in our heads. And you
> know, it's projection. It's the pot calling the kettle black. It's like they were
> characterizing what we were doing as political when in fact every single one
> of their arguments was political. They couldn't address the fact that there
> was no basis for cutoffs [of symptoms in the definition]. (personal interview,
> June 4, 1990)

Proinclusion advocates also identified as political the debates over the
"facts" of PMS and LLPDD. Spitzer acknowledged that the partial success
of the anti-inclusion arguments came from trying to keep the focus on the
scientific evidence or, in this case, on the lack of clear scientific data:

> There were a lot of factual things that were being disputed. You know, "is
> there really any evidence of any effective treatment?" At the time there was
> another strong argument, that there was no value to having the category if
> you didn't have any effective treatments anyway. (personal interview, May
> 23, 1991)

While comparing the earlier APA homosexuality debates (see Bayer 1987)
to the LLPDD controversy, Spitzer stated:

> In 1973 there was no suggestion that 'Gee, if we really study homosexuality
> we can come up with some cure and all our boys [sic] could be saved from
> this thing'. And also there was no biological . . . I mean, the homosexuality
> thing was entirely a debate about value systems. There was no factual dis-
> putes. Whereas with the Late Luteal there were a lot of factual disputes. I

mean, "Are there women who have this and don't have anything else?" That was unclear, but we said yes. Turned out we were right but we didn't really have any evidence. Didn't have any solid evidence. (personal interview, May 23, 1991)

However, for Spitzer, identification of politics behind the uncertainty of the "facts" did not justify exclusion of LLPDD from the DSM-III-R. Just because diagnoses are political does not mean that they cannot be scientific. As he stated: "I enjoy controversy. I love it, so. And I've loved this diagnosis more than the others. I mean, I think it has more to argue for it than the others that were controversial" (personal interview, Robert Spitzer, May 23, 1991, New York City).

This view of science was not shared by one anti-inclusion scientist. A major disappointment expressed by Hamilton was profound disillusionment about the way that "science" was conducted and discussed in the LLPDD controversy. She stated that working on the diagnosis "was a very traumatic experience in terms of my vision of science. . . . It [LLPDD] was not motivated by an interest in science—by finding a real answer to the questions. I guess that was my disappointment. I wanted people to want to understand something about hormones so that we could tell my grandmother whether she should take posthormonal estrogen therapy or not. I mean I wanted a real answer. Not just a fake answer" (personal interview, Jean Hamilton, June 6, 1990).

According to LLPDD critics Parlee and Hamilton, the outcome of biomedical interest in PMS and LLPDD has resulted in greater intrascientific disciplinary competition for jurisdiction over PMS. Tighter control by psychiatrists and biomedical scientists over the definition and scientific research on PMS is the result. Biomedical researchers have successfully incorporated social science and feminist critiques about PMS research and methodology. At the same time, recent biomedical research has restricted research to questions about hormonal changes and other biologically related factors that only biomedically trained M.D.s can answer.

A greater emphasis on mood disorders and cyclical hormonal influences in women's bodies takes PMS out of the realm of therapists, general practitioners, and social scientists, and puts it in the hands of biomedical scientists and psychiatrists. In addition, M.D.s carry greater credibility than social scientists with funding agencies, which results in "conceptual control over what questions will and will not be asked in the research and what methods will be used" (Parlee 1992:6).

In spite of continued resistance by social scientists and general practitioners, LLPDD was generally "welcomed by clinical practitioners as a guide for the psychotherapeutic and pharmacological interventions implemented to relieve the persistent suffering of their clients" (Hood

1992:84). Since no known effective cure exists, doctors and therapists wanted something to give patients—even if it was just a diagnosis. This suggests yet another actor in the science domain and in the construction of LLPDD as a scientific artifact.

As shown in Chapter 1, the pharmaceutical industry began to offer over-the-counter PMS drugs and more PMS-related products in the 1980s. At a time when professional attention was being focused on the creation of LLPDD as a psychiatric diagnosis, total consumer spending in 1984 for menstrual pain relievers including PMS products (and excluding common pain relievers ibuprofen, aspirin, and acetaminophen) was $111,132,000 (Ehrlich 1985:50). If PMS clinics and other treatment prescriptions did not work, then the sales for over-the-counter pharmaceuticals might be put in jeopardy. As an editor of an FDA publication for health professionals wrote in 1983:

> Much is yet to be learned about the monthly cycle women experience. But science increasingly is focusing attention on discovering the physiological basis for the discomfort many women know, and on finding safe and effective ways to relieve these symptoms. (Willis 1983:14)

So, according to gynecologists, the pharmaceutical industry, and government officials, the key to helping women with their PMS was science and more research.

What is the nature of the relationship of PMS-related products to PMS research in the scientific community? One charge was that the diagnosis was created only to secure more funding from pharmaceutical companies or agencies like the NIMH. According to Hamilton: "Drug companies are not going to fund research on this unless we have a diagnosis because they are not going to give you money to test drugs for something that doesn't exist" (Jean Hamilton, personal interview, June 4, 1990). However, the relationship between pharmaceutical companies and the creation of LLPDD was not so simple. One of the most interesting artifacts of the LLPDD controversy was the advertisement for PreMysyn PMS, an over-the-counter PMS drug discussed at the end of Chapter 5. The advertisement appeared in a popular magazine (*People*, June 30, 1986) the same week that the Board of Trustees made their decision about the PMS diagnosis.

Chattem Pharmaceutical's advertisement for PreMysyn PMS represents a challenge to (not support of) the scientific and medical expertise of psychiatrists over PMS. It portrays the psychiatrist's couch, with the words "Premenstrual Tension is not a psychological issue. It is a physical condition." This advertisement could be read as an effort to demarcate the boundary between physical treatment of PMS (which can be treated with products such as PreMysyn PMS) and the "mental" treatment of LLPDD (which has no over-the-counter pharmaceutical products). It directly and not so subtlety suggests to women that physical conditions such as headaches, bloating, and swelling can be taken care of with their products. The text states: "Premenstrual Tension is not in your mind. It's in your body. Use your head. Get to the physical source." The psychiatric couch is not needed to take care of the very physical problems related to PMS. The solution to the PMS problem for women can be found in their product, which contains the FDA-approved combination of an antihistamine, a diuretic, and a pain reliever—as opposed to the APA's product of LLPDD.

In spite of the charge that economic interests of pharmaceutical companies were advanced by the creation of LLPDD, there is not sufficient evidence to indicate that this was the case. Pharmaceutical companies became actors in this domain through the identification of their position by other actors and by advertising their products against the "competition." What can be established is that pharmaceutical companies did increase their sales of PMS-related products in the 1980s. Increased attention to the creation of PMS as a biomedical problem would appear to benefit drug sales.

THE SCIENTIFIC SETTLEMENT OF THE LLPDD CONTROVERSY

The first two parts of this chapter established how and why the sociology of science literature constructed LLPDD as a scientific artifact, and showed how and why debate over the scientific existence of a PMS-related psychiatric diagnosis was highly contested. How was the "truth" and "scientific facts" about PMS and LLPDD eventually settled? In this final section, I argue that "science" itself was ultimately used as a tool for settling the controversy by placing LLPDD in an appendix.

According to Bevins (1990), professional groups that are in positions of power and strength want to close a controversy quickly by claiming to have clear scientific evidence; those that are in weaker positions try to keep the controversy alive by pointing to the lack of clear scientific evidence. This point is well illustrated by debates over the scientific validity of LLPDD and PMS research.

Actors in the entrenched position of power argued that "this *is* science" and that scientific studies are helpful to women by acknowledging the existence of PMS and LLPDD. Proinclusion actors pointed to culturally ingrained notions that suggest that "science" is supposed to be separate from politics. For example, Sally Severino suggested that although little is known about the etiology of PMS: "If we had waited until all the evidence was in, we would never have come up with the staging of heart disease or cancer. We have to begin by labeling, classifying, and defining. This is the way science progresses" (as quoted in Staver 1986b:26). This illustrates how proinclusion scientists were more effectively able to draw upon the "cognitive authority" of science.

Cognitive authority is "the legitimate power (in designated contexts) to define, describe or explain bounded realms of reality" (Gieryn and Figert 1986:67). Thus, in spite of the fact that some anti-inclusion actors also had a measure of "cognitive authority," the image of the proinclusion scientists—representing the NIMH and the APA—carried more weight. Their "interests" were not as apparent or as easily recognized as the anti-inclusion, "feminist" objectors. In other words, they looked more objective, politically neutral, and detached—in short, more scientific.

This appeal to the cultural authority of science was used to demarcate a space for psychiatry in the treatment of women with PMS. Spitzer claimed that the psychiatric diagnosis of LLPDD is "justified in view of the fact that the majority of women who complain to their doctors are more distressed about the psychological than the physical symptoms" (Holden 1986:230). If women are more distressed about psychological symptoms, then psychiatry, the science of the mind, would be the best profession to treat women. Proinclusion actors appealed to our notions about "science" as the great adjudicator. They argued that if disorders are not recognized formally by the psychiatric profession it cannot be treated effectively and that women would suffer as a result (as found in Boxer 1987:82 and Carey 1986:60).

On the opposition side of a scientific controversy, less powerful groups claim that the studies are not "good science." Jasanoff finds this same pattern in the daminozide/Alar controversy, where Uniroyal's strategy was to discredit studies of the opposing view so "as to leave no credible support for the proposition that either daminozide or its metabolite UDMH were carcinogens" (Jasanoff 1987:118). Throughout the LLPDD controversy, opposition forces held to their position that available scientific research does not support inclusion of a PMS-related diagnosis in the DSM-III-R. Hamilton and Alagna argued at the 1986 APA convention debate that the "psychiatric research on premenstrual changes 'has been seriously flawed because of a lack of sufficient controls'" and that "if we're going to have a new diagnosis, we must have objective measures to confirm it. You cannot make this diagnosis based solely on self-reports" (as reported in Staver, 1986a:26).

Lenore Walker, the chair of the Women's Caucus within the American Psychological Association Council of Representatives, stated that the diagnosis of what was called LLPDD emerged "not from a research data base but from a handful of clinical observations" (as quoted in Fisher 1986a). The APA's Committee on Women remained opposed to inclusion even in the Appendix. They argued in their statement that "scientific evidence was still lacking for a premenstrual syndrome diagnosis, considering its potential for stigmatizing women by linking a psychiatric disorder with the menstrual cycle" (as reported in *Psychiatric News*, July 18,1986).

A different strategy of opposition forces was to make the professional scientific controversy into a public controversy. Because opposition forces were not in power, such public attention and controversy delayed decision about LLPDD. The strategy to "go public" with information about possible inclusion of a PMS-related diagnosis worked. LLPDD became the focus of a public science controversy, and opened the possibility for a loss of scientists' control over knowledge and more generally for a loss of the public's faith in science. Public controversies over scientific knowledge reveal that science is political. Expert knowledge of psychiatry was "at risk" in the controversy because of the publicity surrounding the inclusion of LLPDD. The scientific and diagnostic process was exposed as a political process.

Following the June 1986 decision to place the diagnosis in an appendix, Bernardez, the Chair of the Committee on Women, stated that "While I would have preferred to see the diagnoses dropped, I believe it is far better to have them in the appendix than in the text. Now while the proponents try to come up with scientific evidence to support inclusion in the text of DSM-IV, we will have the opportunity to educate our colleagues and the public" about the damaging effects of inclusion in the psychiatric manual (as reported in Staver 1986b:41). This statement nicely supports the assertion by the Committee on Women that scientific evidence about LLPDD did not exist in the first place.

There is however an irony about this anti-inclusion strategy. Although opponents showed that the diagnostic process was political, they held the belief that somehow in the end, science would arrive at the truth about PMS and LLPDD. Spitzer later commented about Hamilton's arguments about the lack of science in the controversy: "[s]he believed it. I don't think it was just a strategy. She really felt the science was very inadequate" (personal interview, May 23, 1991). It was this basic belief in science and its role as the great arbitrator of the world that settled the question about LLPDD. And, in claiming ultimate ownership of LLPDD, the APA Board of Trustees used the established cultural authority of science to effectively settle the controversy.

By including LLPDD in Appendix A of the DSM-III-R as a category in need of "further systematic clinical study and research," the Board of Trustees appealed to lack of scientific data about PMS. Elissa Benedek, APA secretary and member of the Ad Hoc committee, emphasized that "the scientific bases for the controversial disorders are not clear at this point" (as quoted in *Psychiatric News*, July 18, 1986). Speaking for the Board, APA President Robert Pasnau stated:

we are not yet convinced that the scientific evidence, while impressive, is sufficiently strong to warrant inclusion in the text of the manual at this time. But ... [is] of sufficient clinical importance to justify publishing [it] in the appendix to the manual for research and educational purposes. (Press Release of APA dated July 1,1986)

In the case of LLPDD, public rhetoric similar to the "truth will out" device described by Gilbert and Mulkay (1984) settled the dispute. According to Gilbert and Mulkay, the "truth will out" device is a reconciliation mechanism used by individual scientists to cover any inconsistences that evolve when scientists are forced to make a choice about interpretations of the world (1984:110). The device "enables speakers to treat their own views as requiring no justification beyond reference to 'experimental facts,' which are treated as coincident with the real world" (Gilbert and Mulkay 1984:110).

Even though the LLPDD controversy was and is seen as political, its settlement suggests that the "right" decision and "right" representation of the real world were made: that the scientific data did not support inclusion in the main text. This representation also suggests that "science" is supposed to be separate from the political realm. Drawing upon this, the Board of Trustees made a political decision: science and scientific knowledge settled the LLPDD controversy and ultimately politics were and will not be important.

CONCLUSIONS: THE BLACK BOX OF LLPDD

The decision to place LLPDD in an appendix stabilized the artifact and effectively ended the controversy. As Bruno Latour points out, the Board of Trustees (like cyberneticians) drew a "Black Box" around it to show that all you need to know is what precedes and follows from it. The insides are imperceptible. Latour states that constructing a black box around an artifact means that "no matter how controversial their history, how complex their inner workings, how large the commercial or academic networks that hold them in place, only their input and output count" (Latour 1987:3). The final construct of LLPDD was formally created by a panel of experts and now exists "out there in the world" as a scientific fact, a psychiatric diagnosis in the DSM-III-R. Input into this black box is *not* the controversy and objections to its inclusion; rather it is whether or not women have the sufficient and necessary symptoms to qualify for the output—the diagnosis of LLPDD.

A study titled "Late Luteal Phase Dysphoric Disorder in Young Women" was published 3 years after the controversy in the *American Journal of Psy-*

chiatry. It was the first scientific study of LLPDD to make no mention of the controversial nature of the diagnosis. Rather, it gave the explanation that "The recent inclusion of diagnostic criteria in the appendix to DSM-III-R, under the heading of Late Luteal Phase Dysphoric Disorder, has established guidelines for clinicians and researchers that can further systematic research in this area" (Rivera-Tovar and Frank 1990).

LLPDD became a black box and the controversy over the inclusion of LLPDD in DSM-III-R closed. Scientists no longer had to justify their research on PMS or the use of their tools to study it. If you wanted to study the psychiatric manifestations of PMS from 1987 through 1994, you had to go through the American Psychiatric Association's DSM-III-R. As SCOT theorists Pinch and Bijker point out: "Closure in technology involves the stabilization of an artifact and the 'disappearance' of problems. To close a technological 'controversy,' one need not solve the problems in the common sense of that word. The key point is whether the relevant social groups see the problem as being solved" (Pinch and Bijker 1987:44).

According to a former APA president and a noted PMS research from the NIMH, closure is best achieved in the way that the LLPDD controversy was settled. They stated in a 1988 review article: "The use of DSM-III-R criteria for the definition of LLPDD, prospective self-rating measurement instruments, and standardized psychiatric diagnostic tools and the assessment of lifetime and family history of psychiatric disorders are important methodological starting points" (Blumenthal and Nadelson 1988:472).

For those scientists who study PMS, the settlement of the controversy had a positive outcome. Even though the "scientific evidence" about the existence of LLPDD was called into question, the placement of it in an appendix under the heading of "proposed diagnoses in need of further study" made big winners out of the scientists who study PMS. Who benefits by further study of LLPDD? Scientists who conduct the study of PMS and who will accordingly receive grants and other support. The role played by the authority of science in settling the controversy (i.e., the data did not support placement in the main text) diffused any possible negative connections to the professions of science and medicine. According to Law, "[c]losure is achieved when debate and controversy about the form of an artifact is effectively terminated" (Law 1987:111).

The third stage of SCOT is to relate the content of the scientific or technological artifact to the wider sociopolitical milieu. Pinch and Bijker claim that this has not been done in science studies, but is done in technological studies. In this chapter, I have documented and argued that LLPDD is a case where the scientific artifacts are sometimes also technological artifacts. The sociocultural and political situation of different social groups involved in the LLPDD controversy shaped and influenced the meanings given to a scientific artifact. Here is a case of the social construction of scientific and medical facts about PMS and the development of a technical artifact—LLPDD.

NOTES

1.   Interestingly, critiques of PMS studies continue and have not really changed in recent years. For example, in a more recent review of the PMS literature, psychiatrists Blumenthal and Nadelson state that "Despite 50 years of study, there is still surprisingly little known about the epidemiology, etiology, and treatment of menstrually related mood disorders. Lack of systematic research in the past, the presence of many confounding variables, and other methodological problems have complicated the research" (1988:466).

2.   The document was titled "Fact Sheet: Action Alert on Sexism in Psychiatric Diagnoses," which was prepared by Dr. Jean Hamilton. The above quotation appeared under the heading "THE DATA DO NOT SUPPORT A SEPARATE MENTAL DISORDER."

3.   This document was found in the personal archives of Dr. Jean Hamilton at the Institute for Research on Women's Health, Washington, D.C.

4.   According to psychiatrists Blumenthal and Nadelson: "only 20% to 50% of premenstrual complaints are actually confirmed by examination of daily self-reports" (1988:471).

5.   From the text of the PMDD Debate, presented by Dr. Sheryl Alagna, Annual Meeting, American Psychiatric Association, Washington, D.C., May 13, 1986.

III

Settling the Conflict

8

Who Won?
Implications and Conclusions

The construction of a PMS-related diagnosis and its inclusion in the American Psychiatric Association's *Diagnostic and Statistical Manual of Mental Disorders*, Third Edition, Revised (DSM-III-R) have proved to be an interesting case in the history of medical and psychiatric diagnosis. It is much more than that. I have argued in this book that only when the LLPDD is examined through its multiple accountings can one fully begin.to understand what happened and why.

Chapter 3 introduced an ex-post-facto or poststabilization account of the controversy using archival, media, and interview data. This account took the form of a narrative: who was involved, what happened, and when. It is not the only, nor will it be the last word about LLPDD. It is, however, "factual" in the sociological sense that facts are constructed and stabilized claims to knowledge or truth by involved actors. I felt that it was necessary to establish with the reader some kind of shared "reality" about the controversy to avoid an infinite regress of constructions and creations of LLPDD. The narrative is the result of my attempt to create this shared reality in this particular text and context.

Chapter 4 introduced three public accounts of the controversy. The economic account explained the LLPDD controversy as a result of the economic benefits accrued to the APA by revising the DSM-III only 7 years after its publication. The political account pitted feminists against psychiatrists in a battle of power and interests. This account occurred throughout the controversy, and exists today as an available explanation for what happened. The rational account emerged after the controversy was over. The inclusion of LLPDD was "explained" as an inevitable outcome of bureaucratic procedure and scientific truth or method.

If the controversy over LLPDD is read merely as an economic justification, a political compromise with women's and feminist groups or as the progressive refinement of scientific-medical diagnoses, then little insight is gained beyond a blow-by-blow chronology. Only with the trio of socio-logical accounts proposed in Chapter 4—each embedded in a distinctive domain of analysis—will our understanding of the stabilization of LLPDD in the appendix of DSM-III-R be appreciably improved. The ownership of this particular social problem is properly interpreted only when the poli-tics and science surrounding LLPDD are brought together.

Sociologically, LLPDD was not "about" *two* opposing groups and inter-ests—one side proinclusion and the other antiinclusion. Nor was it simply "about" the scientific facts of the matter or "about" how the APA bureau-cratically decides diagnostic policies. Rather, the controversy engaged a much larger and variegated cast of characters. Their interests, strategies, alliances, and goals were more nuanced and more fluid than a simple pro-versus antimodel would suggest. It takes an analysis of three domains of struggle, not one, to expose these subtleties.

Chapters 5, 6, and 7 explored these domains separately, and in depth. In the "health and mental health domain," LLPDD became the site of contests for professional dominance over the control of health and mental health problems. In the "woman domain," LLPDD became part of the struggle over who has authority to define a normal and healthy woman. In the "sci-ence domain," LLPDD became part of a larger struggle for control over de-finitions of "scientific truth" amid public controversy. In each domain, diverse actors with different interests struggled for the definition, owner-ship, and control of PMS.

Not to be lost within these three bounded struggles are the broader so-ciological issues and methodological implications of this study. For exam-ple, throughout the book, I have focused upon the *construction of facts and artifacts* and the *ownership of social problems*, and how these are tied to issues of power and control. LLPDD was deemed an important artifact by differ-ent social actors and groups who engaged in struggle with each other over the right to define and control PMS. Each party claiming control over LLPDD used a distinctive power-base (personal experience, scientific expertise, interests of women, etc.) to justify their authority to define the phenomenon.

Importantly, however, I explicitly reject the kind of reductionistic think-ing expressed in both the realist and interest positions. Is LLPDD a true representation of real, severe emotional symptoms of PMS, or is it a sim-ple case of constructed knowledge based only upon "interests" of certain powerful groups? Neither the realist position nor the interest model *alone* fully explains the multiple realities of LLPDD. Examination of the data in three different domains allows the analyst and the reader to recognize that LLPDD is not *just* about interests, not *just* about power, and not *just* about whether it is a true reflection of the natural world. It is all of these.

The "domain analysis" offered here invites attention to significant and enduring sociological questions: "Who is making these claims and why?" "On what grounds does a certain claim to truth exist?" and "How is this truth determined and settled?" The settlement of controversy certainly reflects the ability of some actors and groups to determine what becomes the accepted view of reality. It also reflects the social, political, and organizational processes through which this occurs. That these same processes can occur in *different* domains of interaction to create different artifacts or outcomes is a measure of the strength of my antireductionistic position.

I have also argued that in the same way that various *participants* can be arrayed in different domains, so too are there distinctive *literatures* in sociology tied to each domain. In this book, previous research in sociology is not brought in to decide the one best account of what happened and why. Instead, concepts and findings from three distinct sociological literatures are themselves part of the story. Each of these literatures constitutes the phenomenon of LLPDD in *irreducibly different ways*.

My most significant methodological conclusion is that "sociology" (as a set of interpretative resources) could *not* adjudicate among several available and plausible accounts of LLPDD; rather, "sociology" *added to their multiplicity*. In the end, the three domains and their distinctive accounts of the inclusion of LLPDD in DSM-III-R are simultaneously constituted by participants in the controversy, by sociological literatures, and by the writer (as she pulled it "all" together).

WHO WON THE LLPDD CONTROVERSY?

In telling people about this controversy, I have found that what they really want to know is "Who won?" and "Why?" I could conclude the analysis at this point by tallying up the outcomes of the settlement, and discussing implications for each group involved. But like everything else in this book, the balance-sheet of winners and losers depends on which account you buy.

If you accept an "economic account" of the controversy, the APA clearly benefited financially from the publication of the DSM-III-R. However, one diagnosis cannot account for the total economic benefits that accrued to the APA from the DSM revision process.

If you accept a "political account" of feminists versus the APA, then maybe "the feminists" won. The APA bowed to "political" pressure and overruled their scientific experts by placing LLPDD in the appendix of the DSM-III-R. On the other hand, individual "feminist" psychiatrists such as Hamilton and Bernardez felt that their careers had been put on hold or were damaged within the APA. If you ask members of the Work Group that revised the DSM, they won in getting it in the DSM-III-R at all but lost on its placement in the appendix. The Ad Hoc Committee won on getting LLPDD in the appendix and in getting physical symptoms added to the diagnosis; they lost on the placement of the other two controversial diagnoses. The APA Committee on Women lost because LLPDD ended up in the DSM-III-R and because it was given a diagnostic code number—but for them placement in the appendix was better than in the main text. The American Psychiatric Association won by creating a temporary research appendix, but lost from adverse publicity generated by the controversy.

It is important to note that adverse publicity affected the political outcome of the controversy for at least one actor in particular, Robert Spitzer. As a result of the controversy over the production of the DSM-III-R, Spitzer was effectively relieved of his position of head of the Work Group to revise future editions of the DSM (see Chapter 9 for more about this). In his own words, the loss of control over the diagnostic process of the APA has "been a very difficult adjustment." Politically, Robert Spitzer appears to be a loser as a result of the APA Board of Trustee's notions "of what's appropriate for the Chairperson to do, how to act, what do you do about controversy and to avoid it" (personal interview, May 23, 1991, New York City).

If you buy the "rational account," there are no winners and losers. Rather, the stabilized outcome is the only logical one, an inevitability "given" by the protocols of scientific truth and bureaucratic procedure. In a rational account, "players" do not have competing interests nor do they fight over LLPDD. Instead, these same players merely feed the best scientific studies through the machinery of the DSM revision process—and out comes the new diagnosis (no struggle at all).

In the health domain of analysis, the outcome was a compromise between gynecologists and psychiatrists. Psychiatrists would not need to make gynecological diagnoses and gynecologists would not need to make psychiatric diagnoses. Both medical specialties were satisfied, except for some gynecologists who objected to a psychiatric diagnosis of PMS on grounds that it was *only* a physical disorder and not a psychiatric one.

Within the psychiatric profession, victory depends on which segment of the APA is considered. In terms of Robert Spitzer and the Work Group, there were small victories in getting the diagnosis in the appendix (versus no diagnosis at all). They succeeded in getting a code assigned to the diagnosis. At the same time, neither the Work Group nor the LLPDD Advisory Committee expected the fierce opposition to the diagnosis, and their being overruled within the APA hierarchy could be seen as a major loss.

For the American Psychiatric Association, there were small defeats due to the loss of organizational control over the DSM revision process—too many other players were let in the room. Perhaps because of this, Spitzer was effectively fired from the Work Group and a new head was chosen to revise DSM-IV. The APA has decided to take greater control of the DSM revision process. For members of the APA Committee on Women, the results of the controversy were somewhat damaging: the two Committee on Women members that spearheaded the opposition (Bernardez and Hamilton) have both effectively quit their participation in the APA, and they feel "blackballed" professionally because of their opposition.

For the nonpsychiatric professionals who opposed the diagnosis, the settlement can be seen as a partial victory. Partial, because the American Psychological Association and the National Association of Social Workers continued to oppose any form of the premenstrual diagnosis in the DSM. However, as a result of their opposition to the diagnosis, the American Psychological Association has secured representation on the Committee to Revise DSM-III-R. For the majority of mental health professionals who opposed the inclusion of LLPDD in any form, the settlement was far from positive.

In the woman domain of analysis, there was a small victory for women in terms of placement of LLPDD in the appendix, and in creating a coalition effective in lobbying the APA. This coalition cut across social and professional boundaries, which contributed much to the successful challenge to get the three controversial diagnoses placed in the appendix. Success was partially achieved in the Board of Trustees' decision, which upheld their arguments that scientific data did not support inclusion.

Although "professional advocates" such as the Committee on Women and the American Psychological Association continued to fight on their behalf, women with PMS who wrote to the APA and signed petitions protesting inclusion appeared to be silenced by the resulting settlement. Inclusion of the diagnosis in the DSM-III-R anywhere signaled defeat for these women who would be subject to the label of having a "mental illness." It is these women who stood to lose the most from the settlement and from publicity generated by the controversy over LLPDD. Early indications from clinical studies suggest that although women cannot be "officially" diagnosed with LLPDD, they are being given this diagnosis in conjunction with other diagnoses such as major depression or borderline personality disorder (personal communication, Bernice Pescosolido). The reality for these women is that the diagnosis of LLPDD is being given to them by health care professionals and is now found on their psychiatric records and charts.

In the science domain, women and feminist groups experienced a huge loss in terms of their faith in "science," and their growing distrust of the APA as neutral proponent of the scientific study of mental disorders. Whereas Robert Spitzer has been involved in many political disputes over diagnoses—and understands the nature of the beast—I think that the Women's Committee of the APA, along with other feminist and professional challengers, believed that "good science" would be enough to settle the issue.

Large gains were made by the APA in placing the diagnosis in the appendix; it makes it appear as if science and not politics will settle the future of LLPDD. Because the Board of Trustees effectively postponed the ultimate decision about LLPDD, the APA won out by getting the controversy to die out for at least 4 years, on grounds that more scientific research would eventually remove lingering doubts and ambiguities.

For scientists who study PMS, the controversy and its settlement were a positive thing. Even though the "scientific evidence" about the existence of LLPDD was called into question, the placement of it under the heading "proposed diagnoses in need of further study" guaranteed more funding for—and increased attention to—PMS-related phenomena. Who benefits by further study of LLPDD? Scientists who conduct the study of PMS and who will receive grants to conduct that research.

The big winner in the science domain was LLPDD: through the controversy, it became FACT. If you (like authors in SSK and SCOT who constituted LLPDD as part of the science domain) believe that nonhuman actors have existences, then LLPDD is the real winner—because it came into being. Still, the settlement of the controversy was only temporary. Decisions made in 1985 and 1986 by the APA Board of Trustees inevitably resulted in the need for yet another decision when revisions DSM-IV were made. LLPDD became a black box but for how long? The Afterword (Chapter 9) explores what happened to LLPDD in the DSM-IV and why it happened the way it did.

9

Afterword:
DSM-IV and the Controversy Revisited

> When the same diagnosis, then called 'late luteal phase dysphoric disorder,' first was listed in the handbook's appendix in 1986, it caused a furor, with major medical and women's groups opposed. Now, with the psychiatrists' deciding to keep the disorder in the appendix and take the further step of listing it in the main text with depressive disorders, anger, controversy and threats of lawsuits have be reignited. (Lehman 1993:33)

In the course of investigating the LLPDD controversy, I have learned that scientific and medical decisions never proceed smoothly or as predicted. This is what makes for an interesting study to sociologists and historians. For example, in 1985, Robert Spitzer did not think that there would be opposition to what became LLPDD. Many people never would have thought that a PMS-related diagnosis would be in the official psychiatric manual. But LLPDD *was* listed in the appendix of DSM-III-R, and the preceding chapters of this book document how and why this one controversy can be interpreted as consisting of three different ownership claims to three different artifacts.

More importantly for this afterword, the focus shifts to how and why a premenstrually-related disorder is now listed in the main text of the manual's latest revision, DSM-IV. There were many twists and turns to the PMS/DSM-IV controversy (American Psychiatric Association 1994). This afterword serves as an update to the ongoing controversy over PMS and the DSM. But it also shows how the settlement of LLPDD in DSM-III-R and the three ownership claims to it (professional, gendered, and scientific) shaped the events that followed. The more things change, the more they stay the same.

A NARRATIVE OF THE DEVELOPMENT OF THE DSM-IV

I need to provide you with another story or narrative. This time the story is that of the development of the DSM-IV and the reintroduction of the diagnosis once again named Premenstrual Dysphoric Disorder (PMDD).[1] Important elements in my narrative include the story of how shifting allegiances, new players, new drug treatments such as the use of the antidepressant Prozac, and the settlement of LLPDD in DSM-III-R all played a role in the resettlement of PMDD in the DSM-IV. However, to fully understand the development and production of the DSM-IV, we must have a sociohistorical understanding of the events and controversy over LLPDD and the DSM-III-R, which were documented in the earlier chapters of this book. In particular, the professional, gendered, and scientific ownership claims made in the DSM-III-R controversy continued to play important roles in the DSM-IV controversy.

In 1988, only 1 year after the publication of DSM-III-R, the APA Board of Trustees established a work group to construct the DSM-IV. The stated reason for the revision was that the DSM-IV needed to be consistent in coding and terminology with revisions of the *International Classification of Diseases* manual (ICD-10) scheduled for publication in the early 1990s by the World Health Organization. The timing of the revision with the ICD and so soon after the publication of DSM-III-R was consistent with the previous DSM revision processes. What was not consistent was the selection of a new chair to head the DSM-IV Task Force.

As indicated in Chapter 8, Robert Spitzer's role in DSM business dramatically changed with the development of DSM-IV. Spitzer was central to the story of the development of DSM-III and DSM-III-R (see Bayer 1987). But Spitzer was relegated to the sidelines in DSM-IV. In my interview with him in 1991, he stated his feelings about being replaced as chair of the DSM Task Force: "Well, I'm involved but I'm not in charge of it. I'm not leading the troops. . . . How do I feel? Terrible" (personal interview, New York City, May 23, 1991). In organizational lingo, Spitzer was named a "Special Advisor" to the Task Force and some of its subcommittees. But he was not in charge of the revision process.[2]

The new Chair of the Task Force to develop DSM-IV was Allen Frances. Frances may have been the perfect candidate; he has great academic and clinical credentials. At the time of his selection, he was a psychiatry professor at Cornell University Medical School and identified himself as a "clinician."[3] He was interested and involved in the issues of psychiatric diagnosis, but was also trained in psychoanalytic theory. He was also no stranger to diagnostic controversy—he was part of the group of psychiatrists who had proposed the inclusion of Masochistic Personality Disorder in DSM-III-R. But controversy was not wanted in the DSM-IV.

It quickly became apparent in my meetings with APA officials and in my interviews with Spitzer, Hamilton, and Severino that the linkage of words "controversy" and the "DSM-IV" was to be avoided—at all costs. One of the ways in which the APA ensured this was to take more organizational control over the DSM-IV revision process. Harold Pincus, a Deputy Medical Director of the APA (Director of Research Division), was appointed Vice-Chair of the Task Force. A separate research director (Thomas Widiger) was also appointed.

Another way that the APA tried to keep any controversy over DSM-IV to a minimum was to state explicitly that any decisions about the manual were to be based upon data and not politics. As foreshadowed in the nature of the settlement of LLPDD, APA officials stressed that science—not politics or individual psychiatrists—would form the basis of the DSM-IV. Having learned from previous controversies and deciding that public controversies harmed the image of psychiatry as scientific medicine, Allen Frances and APA officials publicly stressed the empirical and scientific process of DSM-IV development (Frances et al. 1989, 1991; Pincus et al. 1992). Early publications about the revision process stated that all decisions would be "empirically based." Frances and members of the committee wrote:

> The Task Force does not expect to completely eliminate controversy from the DSM-IV but is doing its best to direct persons back to a quiet consideration of the evidence rather than a loud expression of their personal views. (Frances et al. 1991:411)

According to its new developers, the DSM-IV revision process would be a three-stage (and scientific) process: (1) reviews of published literature, (2) analyses of collected but not yet analyzed data, and (3) field trials (funded in Part by the MacArthur Foundation and sponsored by NIMH and others) designed to "bridge the boundary between clinical research and clinical practice by determining how well suggestions for change that are derived from clinical research findings apply in clinical practice" (APA 1994:xix).

The manner in which the revisions to DSM-IV were organized and proceeded gives us hints about the way in which the question of LLPDD was handled in the DSM-IV. Was LLPDD to be included in the DSM-IV or dropped as a diagnostic/research category? If it was included, would it be in the main text or another appendix? Would it be given a code number or not? In the words of the DSM-IV writers, new diagnoses would be carefully scrutinized:

> On the other hand, new diagnoses that are subject to controversy and/or possible misuse will require especially strong empirical support. Insofar as possible, we will attempt to avoid controversies by including only those new diagnoses that command widespread empirical and clinical support. (Pincus et al., 1992:115)

Keeping controversy to a minimum and holding the line of the proliferation of new diagnoses were the key issues facing the developers of DSM-IV and eventually the LLPDD/PMDD advisory group appointed to derive an "expert" consensus. Controversy was to be avoided and the way to do this was to make a decision based upon science and empirical data. Sounds easy. Based upon what happened with DSM-III-R, we know it was not.

THE LLPDD/PMDD WORK GROUP

The committee that would decide the fate of LLPDD's status in the DSM-IV was carefully selected. Judith Gold, a clinician and PMS researcher at the University of Nova Scotia, was appointed the chair of the LLPDD (later the PMDD work group). Its members included three scientists who previously served on the LLPDD Advisory Committee on DSM-III-R: Barbara Parry, Sally Severino, and Jean Endicott. Nada Stotland (then Chair of the APA Committee on Women) was the final member. Ellen Frank, who along with Gold was a member of the DSM-IV Task Force, was listed as a consultant to the group. In 1990, according to LLPDD opponent Jean Hamilton, it looked as if the advisory committee was once again stacked in favor of making this a full-force diagnosis in the main text:

> So they got this woman named July Gold. She's very even handed and well regarded and very cautious and stuff. She's the chair but either she was given a biased committee or she chose a biased committee because who she appointed as the main leaders with her were Barbara Parry and Sally Severino, representing one side of the debate. Now how can you even pretend, I mean in the law there's a phrase called whether something is blushable. It's blushable if you can go up before the judge and make this argument without like turning red. I don't think that her chairing this committee with one side of the debate is blushable. It's such a fantastic kind of process they go through. (personal interview, June 4, 1990 Washington, D.C.)

By 1991, Robert Spitzer predicted that the way the committee was composed would eventually recommend full inclusion in the DSM-IV:

> So, the question is what is this Committee going to do. Now, it's clear, at least to me, that three people on that Committee and if you include Ellen Frank, that's four, believe there's no doubt that this thing should be conceptualized as a disorder and that it should be upgraded. Nada Stotland, who is going off the Women's Committee, though I guess she'll probably stay on this Committee, I'm sure because of her political perspective, she's going to say let's leave it in the appendix. And then I guess Judy Gold, I don't know what she'll do. (personal interview, May 23, 1991 New York City)

A year later, PMS researcher Mary Parlee, who served as an Advisor to the PMDD Committee and participated in the campaign opposing its inclusion in the DSM-IV, predicted:

> I predict LLPDD **will** be included in DSM-IV for scientific reasons—not in the school-book sense of science (in which we as feminists often put too much faith), but in the demystified understanding of scientific practices that has come out of the past 15 years of science studies. (Parlee 1992:106–107)

In spite of the many early predictions about the future of LLPDD in the DSM-IV, the mission of the work group was clear (at least to its members): "The working group was charged with reaching a consensus, and 'I was quite hopeful that we could,' says Ellen Frank, a psychologist who directs the University of Pittsburgh School of Medicine's depression prevention program. 'It was an extremely reasonable, thoughtful group of women'" (as quoted in Span 1993:C2). According to Gold, the chair of the group, their task was the following:

> A work group was formed within this task force to study the diagnosis of LLPDD and to determine whether sufficient data existed in research studies to justify its classification as a mental disorder or, if not, whether it should remain in the appendix of DSM-IV to be studied further. The basic issues to be examined were the validity and clinical usefulness of this proposed new disorder as described in the appendix of the DSM-III-R; that is, was there a clinically significant mental disorder associated with the menstrual cycle, and could it be distinguished from other mental disorders? (Gold 1994:175)

The work group set about the arduous task of wading through the results of the data reanalysis project about LLPDD and PMS:

> The analysis showed that the prevalence of LLPDD varied depending upon which scoring method was used.... Based upon this data reanalysis, the phenomenology of LLPDD was changed.... The name LLPDD was also changed to premenstrual dysphoric disorder (PMDD). (Gold 1994:177)

An often quoted figure in the debate that only about 5% of all menstruating women would be eligible for this diagnosis appears to be based upon Rivera-Tovar and Frank's (1990) study in the *American Journal of Psychiatry* (mentioned in Chapter 7 as the article that helped "black box" LLPDD as a scientific artifact). Sally Severino acknowledged the difficulty of the PMDD situation when the interests of "women's rights" and psychiatric "nosology" seem to collide. Her solution is not to abandon this challenge but to engage in the struggle: "[w]e must negotiate a name and a process for understanding the condition that is acceptable to all those threatened by the change, while not sacrificing the goal of understanding and helping women" (Severino 1994:223). For Severino, the process that the work group members followed was once again the way in which good science proceeds: "PMS and LLPDD must be named and defined. That has been the focus of the DSM process, both for DSM-III-R . . . and DSM-IV. Select a name. Describe the condition in terms of symptoms, signs in manifest behavior, and conscious experience of it, both by the woman and the significant others in her life. Then the condition can be studied" (Severino 1994:224). This is what the PMDD committee did, but the results proved more perplexing than expected.

WHAT'S IN A NAME?—REVISITED

One of the more interesting things about the DSM-III-R story was how the name of the diagnosis went through its many changes and how the APA leaders tried to account for the changes in light of scientific and precise medical terminology. There were also public statements and acknowledgments made by APA leaders about the possibility that the term "Premenstrual Dysphoric Disorder" would stigmatize women. So, the question arises: *Why was the name changed from Late Luteal Phase Dysphoric Disorder (LLPDD) back to Premenstrual Dysphoric Disorder (PMDD)?* In the quotations above by Gold and Severino, the name change is taken as a given byproduct of the way in which the revision process occurred. The issues of precision and stigmatization have fallen away. One of the stated reasons for publishing the DSM-IV so soon after DSM-III-R (7 years) was to be compatible (as required by the U.S. treaty with the World Health Organization) with the International Classification of Diseases (ICD-10). The only justification that I can find "in print" for the name change is the following:

> The older term *premenstrual tension,* coined by Frank (1931), is included in the ICD nomenclature under 'Diseases of the Genitourinary System (N00-N99): N94: Pain and other conditions associated with female genital organs and the menstrual cycle'. (as quoted in Gold 1994:175)

In addition, according to a memo written by Gold (and forwarded to opponent Paula Caplan), the name change would "reflect data showing that the etiology of the symptom pattern may not be due to the hormones of the luteal phase" (as quoted in Caplan 1995:136). However, if part of the stated and public reason for the revision to take place was ICD-10 compatibility (for coding and data collection purposes), then it would make sense from a nomenclature point of view to return to use of the name premenstrual dysphoric disorder.

Having lived and breathed this material for so many years and having talked to many mental health professionals, my conclusion is that the name was changed because most practicing mental health professionals do not know what "late luteal phase dysphoric disorder" means . . . the severe dysphoria associated with the premenstruum. Thus, I believe that the name change back to PMDD was partially done to make the diagnosis more accessible to potential DSM-IV users. As PMDD critic Paula Caplan (whose role is explored in greater detail later in the chapter) explains:

> The double-barreled power of the LLPDD label was that in two ways it made it harder to criticize, because it made it harder even for most therapists—not to mention the public—to understand. In the first place, few people would readily recognize that Late Luteal Phase Dysphoric Disorder was a fancy name for PMS, making it likely that few would ever even wonder whether this new category needed thoughtful examination. In the second place, the new label gave the impression of great scientific precision, since it seemed that one was no longer dealing with some vague, general time before menstrual bleeding began but rather with some apparently highly specific, clearly identifiable few days in the *late* part of the *luteal* phase of the cycle. (Caplan 1995:92)

Once again the issue of naming this created psychiatric disorder was of great importance to the builders of the DSM. But unlike the DSM-III-R, there seems to be no publicly stated reason for the change back to Premenstrual Dysphoric Disorder—a name with the built-in possibility of stigmatizing all women.

DIVISIONS WITHIN THE PMDD COMMITTEE

The work group was also given the task of examining the research and diagnostic criteria for the PMS-related diagnosis. Were the symptoms and other criteria for Late Luteal Phase Dysphoric Disorder in the DSM-III-R sufficient, or were new criteria based upon the latest scientific studies needed? This is when controversy heated up—not as a public controversy but rather as controversy and contention within the PMDD Committee itself. One media article reports a significant shift in the nature of the positions held within the group:

> This was a collegial group, but by last summer, as talk turned to what the group should recommend to the task force overseeing all DSM-IV revisions, the divergence of opinion was clear. At the final session in Washington last winter, some group members argued from moving PMDD into the Diagnostic and Statistical Manual as a recognized diagnosis and others urged that it

be deleted or relegated to the appendix, pending much more information. It was a hung jury. (Span 1993:C2)

Sally Severino was in charge of the analysis of the data about LLPDD. According to reports in the press, she

> was disturbed by her analysis of data—1,089 women's records of 2,106 menstrual cycles—collected from patients seeking PMS treatment. Depending on what criteria were used, the proportion who would receive a PMDD diagnosis showed unsettling variation—from 14 percent to 45 percent. 'I felt we did not have a reliable method for making this diagnosis,' Severino says. 'There is a condition that women report having; I don't know what the condition is.' She wanted to keep PMDD in the appendix. (Span 1993:C2)

This represented a shift in her position from wanting LLPDD in the main text of the manual. The reason for this shift in thinking is suggested in the following portrayal:

> Dr. Sally K. Severino, another committee member and a psychiatrist at New York Hospital-Cornell Medical Center, Westchester Division, says the disorder belongs in the book's appendix, as it is now, listed only as worthy of further study. (Lehman 1993:36)

This is a case of where the appendix's function of encouraging further studies of diagnosis has led to doubt by one of the original supporters. As another report indicates, Severino

> would have preferred to 'leave things as they were' in the previous edition, published in 1987. There, a similar condition, called 'late luteal phase dysphoric disorder', or LLPDD, lurked in the limbo of the appendix. 'I see no point in changing the name again,' says Severino. 'There have been 15 names already. It just confuses people.' Moreover, she says, 'this new classification puts an emphasis on depression, rather than keeping an open mind.' Severino supported the initial decision to put a premenstrual disorder in the manual, and is convinced that having LLPDD in print for the past seven years 'has stimulated research and encouraged physicians to think about mental functioning. It did all we hoped it would.' (as quoted in Vines 1994:12–13)

Nada Stotland, representing the APA's Committee on Women on the PMDD Advisory Committee, was portrayed as one of the strongest public voices against the inclusion of the diagnosis anywhere in the DSM-IV (but above all not in the main text) as seen in the following:

> Gold's committee, however, was far from unanimous. Another member, Dr. Nada L. Stotland, a University of Chicago psychiatrist, believes the listing

may harm women and stunt research into the effects of the menstrual cycle. (Lehman 1993:36)

Stotland was seen in the press accounts as "probably focused most on the socio-cultural questions. 'Women endure more abuse, more inequality and more disrespect than men, and they're not supposed to show any anger about it,' she says. 'It could be that over the course of the normal menstrual cycle there is a greater tendency to manifest behaviors which are quite appropriate, under the circumstances, but which the woman herself finds very disturbing'" (Span 1993:C2).[4]

Another committee member, Barbara Parry, went on record in the same article as taking "issue with" the solutions of omitting or keeping in an appendix: "To me, that message is 'We're not really sure this exists. We don't have the confidence to put this in the body [of the manual]. It's no-man's land.' She wanted PMDD formally recognized and thought the opposition more politically than scientifically motivated" (as quoted in Span 1993:C2). Her opinion was apparently shared by committee member Jean Endicott: "I thought there was very strong, full evidence to include it fully in the [text of the DSM],.... We actually know more about this condition than we know about some of the other conditions in the nomenclature" (as quoted in Span 1993:C2).

This posed a very big problem. If the task force composed of PMS experts could not form an expert consensus about LLPDD's nature, what would happen to its placement in the DSM-IV? Span reports that

> Had it come to a ballot, the group would probably have voted 3 to 2, with the chair abstaining, to include PMDD in the new manual. But given its more difficult assignment—consensus—the group had to report to the task force that it had reached an impasse. (Span 1993:C2)

Robert Spitzer gave me the following prediction about this possibility in 1991:

> Now, Alan Francis has already said, he said at a meeting here, at a meeting in New Orleans, that if the Committee votes three to two, that is if it's not a unanimous vote he would certainly not be in favor of upgrading its status. I think that's outrageous because the real issue is not the Committee, three to two, particularly when you pick two people who are not even experts in the area. The real issue is what do the experts in the area think and then the second issue is, okay they may want it upgraded but maybe there's still a lot of opposition so you have to find out but I object to the idea that a Committee has to unanimously vote. (personal interview, May 23, 1991, New York City)

As the various reports in the media and the publicly reported statements by the work group members suggest, no consensus was reached within the PMDD committee but a solution was still needed.

THE SETTLEMENT (THE IRONY AND THE CONSEQUENCES)

It is ironic that with all the emphasis on expert consensus and empirical research surrounding the DSM-IV, these goals fell by the wayside in light of the controversy over PMDD. Robert Spitzer was prescient in his observation in 1991 that even though the DSM-IV people were publicly trying to rely only upon empirical evidence, in the end politics would rule out. He stated then that

> My own prediction is that when final decisions are made about DSM-IV, they will still be based primarily on expert consensus, rather than on data, as was the case with the DSM-III and DSM-III-R. (Spitzer 1991:294)

As a result of the disagreements and lack of "expert consensus" by the appointed PMS experts on the PMDD advisory board, the decision about PMDD's placement in the DSM-IV fell to two nonexperts in the PMS field [two psychiatrists on the DSM-IV Work Group (see Span 1993; Caplan 1995)]. Alan Francis appointed two Work Group members (initially not identified to the public) to settle the dispute. Press accounts report that

> Even the American Psychiatric Association's own committee composed to deal with the disorder was so divided that it gave up trying to form a consensus and handed over its working papers to other psychiatrists to resolve the question. (Lehman 1993:33)

An *APA Monitor* article reported that

> The work group was so divided, in fact, they had to call on two outside reviewers—Nancy Andreason, MD, and A. John Rush, MD, both members of the DSM task force—to make the final decision on how to hand the diagnosis. (De Angelis 1993:32)

But in this case, the "experts" were psychiatrists with expertise in depression and schizophrenia—not PMS. Once again, nonexpert psychiatrists ultimately made the decision about the scientific merits of including a PMS-related diagnosis in the DSM. The "research criteria" for PMDD would stay in a research appendix—Appendix B of DSM-IV. But PMDD also receives prominent mention in the main text of DSM-IV as a mood disorder: "Depressive Disorder Not Otherwise Specified." PMDD is the first diagnosis listed in this category with a paragraph of explanation about the diagnosis and the reference to the page number for the "suggested research criteria" (American Psychiatric Association 1994:350). According to Gold, this would provide "recognition to the small number of women who do suffer from severe, incapacitating dysphoria premenstrually" (as quoted in Cotton 1993:14).

But if we are really keen observers and consumers of mental health politics, we know that it does more than just recognize these women. It classifies them as having a legitimate (and legitimated) psychiatric disorder. Women are given this diagnosis with the official code number 311; it is reimbursable by third party insurance payments and it is recorded on a woman's medical chart. This points to a very important distinction made about the way in which criteria for Premenstrual Dysphoric Disorder are presented in the DSM-IV. The term "diagnostic" criteria would imply that an actual diagnosis is made; rather, the criteria for Premenstrual Dysphoric Disorder are presented under the heading "Research criteria for premenstrual dysphoric disorder," which would imply that PMDD is "not-quite" an "official" diagnosis . . . except when listed under Depressive Disorder Not Otherwise Specified.[5] As PMDD critic Carol Tavris notes:

> The list of criteria for diagnosing PMDD gives the game away. . . . How does this list differ from the popular concept of PMS? (Not at all.) What is to prevent psychiatrists from overdiagnosing this 'disorder,' as they already do? Where is the stipulation that this diagnosis must depend on measuring a woman's hormone levels, to separate a woman with PMDD from one whose problem is depression? (Tavris 1993:B7)

She concludes that

> In bestowing its self-serving approval to this label, the psychiatric Establishment feeds the prejudice that women's hormones, but not men's, are a cause of mental illness. (Tavris 1993:B7)

In addition, whether PMDD is truly a distinct or an underlying depressive disorder is still in question. Gold suggests that cross-listing PMDD under a depressive disorder fits some women's needs:

> `There is a very tiny number of women who have a mental disorder. They are severely depressed and would be recognized as depressed no matter what,' says Gold. 'The only difference is that is occurs only part of the month.' (Lehman 1993:36)

However, other PMS scientists disagree and wonder if PMS manifests the symptoms of some other underlying depression or is a distinct depression. PMS physician Michelle Harrison is quoted as saying that "some women with incapacitating premenstrual depression are in reality suffering from an underlying depression that is magnified in the week or two before menses. She points out that many chronic conditions in women—such as epilepsy and asthma—worsen during the premenstrual period" (Lippert 1994:94). Gold however "argues that premenstrual depression is not related to some underlying depression. She amplifies: 'A number of carefully done studies show that women with severe premenstrual depression are typically very competent and mentally healthy in the first two weeks of their cycles, and then behave like a clinically depressed person for some part of the two weeks before menstruation'" (Lippert 1994:94).

In yet another ironic shift, the new director of the Institute for Research on Women's Health (the office where the fight against the inclusion of LLPDD in the DSM-III-R was led) is portrayed in the press as supporting the notion of a uniquely premenstrual depression:

> Some experts recommend that women who suffer from *severe* premenstrual depression seek counseling and, if necessary, discuss the possibility of taking antidepressants with their therapists. All three major classes of antidepressants—the serotonin-specific drugs, such as Prozac; the tricyclics, such as Elavil; and the monoamine-oxidase inhibitors (M.A.O.I.s), such as Nardil—can be helpful, says Margaret Jensvold, M.D., director of the Institute for Research on Women's Health in Washington, DC. (Lippert 1994:94)

Jensvold is then quoted as saying that she "thinks that P.M.D.D.'s entry in the D.S.M. will stimulate needed research on the subject. Her reply to the argument that the diagnosis will be used against women? 'I'm strongly opposed to the stereotyping and stigmatization of women.' But that's not a valid reason to be against a diagnosis. One should be against the misuse of the diagnosis in a way that stigmatizes women" (Lippert 1994:95). Stigmatization against women was one of the most important arguments used against the inclusion of LLPDD in the DSM-III-R, but took on lesser importance in the DSM-IV controversy. I believe that one of the reasons why this is the case is connected to the rise of prescription drugs used to "effectively" treat women and PMS.

PMDD AND THE DRUG CONNECTION

The issue of having pharmaceuticals that work in women's PMS treatments makes the PMDD controversy different than the LLPDD controversy. Prozac and the other drugs were not available for prescription to women with PMS in 1985–1987. One of the main (and more effective) arguments against the inclusion of LLPDD was "how can we have a diagnosis when there are no efficacious treatments for this disorder"? By 1994, this issue had changed. Gold is quoted as being worried "that if psychiatrists and physicians aren't knowledgeable about P.M.D.D., women with the disorder won't be given therapy and/or antidepressants—which, she believes, can be very helpful" (Lippert 1994:95). The debate over drugs harkens back to the issues of professional dominance among mental health professionals that were so important in the DSM-III-R controversy. Using antidepressants in treating PMDD makes sense if women believe it works; it also makes sense that only medical doctors can prescribe antidepressants. Other mental health professionals have to refer their clients to a physician for this kind of treatment. This point is seen in the following quotation:

> Some psychologists contend that the psychiatric association's major motivation in creating the diagnosis is the bottom line. One clue that that's the case is that 'the DSM people have not claimed psychotherapy as a solution' to such problems, according to Dr. Caplan. Instead, they tout antidepressants, the effectiveness is hotly debated, she said. (as quoted in De Angelis 1993:33)

Recent studies reported in the *Journal of the American Medical Association* (*JAMA*) and *The New England Journal of Medicine* are some of the first to report favorable effectiveness rates (50% improvement of symptoms) of the antidepressant drug fluoxetine (known as Prozac) and the antianxiety prescription alprozolam (known as Xanax) when compared to placebo or progesterone treatments.[6] To medicate or not to medicate with these very powerful prescription drugs is an issue that women, their physicians, and mental health professionals now have to consider. With the expense associated with these drugs, many women are less concerned with the stigmatizing label of having a psychiatric disorder from the DSM-IV than with getting the some sort of reimbursement from their insurance for their diagnosed PMS.

THE OPPOSITION FORCES

So far, the story I have told of PMDD and the DSM-IV may have given you the impression that the action took place solely within the APA and the PMDD Work Group with mostly scientific and professional issues involved. This was far from the case. Like the LLPDD and the DSM-III-R controversy, this was a very public controversy. Although the APA leaders and Allen Frances wanted to keep any controversy over the DSM-IV to a minimum, once again the gendered issues of "Women and PMS" took center stage. Unlike the DSM-III-R, the primary ringleader(s) of the opposition forces did not come from within the psychiatric profession but came from Paula Caplan, a psychologist from the University of Toronto.

Caplan is the author of the book *The Myth of Women's Masochism* (1985) and is an expert in the mental health field. Caplan became involved in diagnostic issues and the DSM revision process in 1985 in the controversy surrounding the proposed diagnosis of "Masochistic Personality Disorder"—later changed to the name "Self-Defeating Personality Disorder" and included with LLPDD in Appendix A of the DSM-III-R. This was the same diagnosis originally proposed by Allen Frances, who later chaired the DSM-IV creation process. As an expert and as a feminist scholar, Caplan was heavily involved in fighting the inclusion of this diagnosis and LLPDD and the other diagnosis seen as harmful to women.

Whereas many of the LLPDD opposition leaders within psychiatry burned out and dropped out of the DSM battles, Caplan stayed with it and continued to fight against what she believed was deliberate and harmful misdiagnosis of women by the American Psychiatric Association and the DSM. Due to her experience in fighting the DSM-III-R battles, Caplan continued to write, talk, and publish about the DSM and the controversial diagnoses related to women (1991, 1995; Caplan et al. 1992). She was even appointed by Allen Frances to serve as a consultant to the Self-Defeating Personality Disorder subcommittee and an adviser to the LLPDD/PMDD subcommittee (Caplan 1995:111).[7] As one reporter indicated:

> Caplan has been a gadfly buzzing around the APA since the last re-tooling of the Diagnostic and Statistical Manual in the mid-'80s. She was among the advisers to the working group on PMDD this round, resigned when she felt her counsel was being ignored, and started cranking up the opposition last winter when the task force decided to recommend including the disorder in DSM-IV. (Span 1993:C2)

Caplan used similar types of opposition tactics and arguments against the inclusion of a PMS-related diagnosis in the DSM-IV to those that were used against LLPDD in the DSM-III-R. She gave lectures, collected names on petitions, and wrote articles (Caplan et al. 1992) debating the inclusion of PMS in the DSM. One journalist concluded that

> Caplan launched an effective media campaign, generating dozens of articles and culminating in a 'Donahue' show frighteningly, if misleadingly, titled 'Psychiatrists Want to Classify Women with PMS as Crazy'. (Span 1993:C2)

Interestingly, Caplan was also able to make effective use of an increasingly popular new technology, the internet. Caplan used electronic mail to reach a large number of people quickly (especially academic feminists with research and political interests in the subject matter). For example, the following post from Caplan appeared on the Women's Studies Electronic Discussion Group and was then forwarded to a Science and Technology Studies Discussion Group:

> I am a psychologist at the University of Toronto and Ontario Institute for Studies in Education. Seven years ago, the American Psychiatric Association proposed three deeply anti-woman categories of mental disorder for its handbook of mental disorders (the DSM), which is extremely influential in deciding all over the world who is defined as normal. Anyway, as you may know, these proposed categories pathologized women. Some of us organized a petition and letter campaign aimed at keeping the categories out, and we had some limited success. Now they are revising the handbook, and though it looks like our efforts at keeping Self-defeating Personality Disorder out (it's the one that blames women for their unhappiness, says they really enjoy it, etc.) have almost succeeded, they are probably going to include Premenstrual Syndrome AS A PSYCHIATRIC DISORDER (not just as some mood or behavior or physical changes that happen to some women before their periods, but A MENTAL ILLNESS)—they plan to include it, and the deadline is just about three weeks away. What they do tend to worry about is the media and public pressure. I have written a one-page info sheet and petition that I'd love to get to as many women and women's groups as possible. How would I go about using your network (WMST-L) for that? And is that appropriate? (Caplan, e-mail transmission dated February 23, 1993)

The information sheet and petition was included on the Women's Studies file list, which could be retrieved electronically.

As a result of this kind of attention getting, the same groups that protested about LLPDD the lack of scientific evidence and the diagnosis being stigmatizing to all women in 1986, protested once again in 1993. The APA's Committee on Women, American Psychological Association, the National Women's Health Network, the Boston Women's Health Book Collective, and the National Organization for Women all formally registered a protest with the American Psychiatric Association over the possible inclusion of PMDD in the DSM-IV. The newsletter of the American Psychological Association reported:

> In an April 20 letter to Judith Gold, MD, who chaired the work group, APA Chief Executive Officer Raymond D. Fowler, PhD, wrote, 'Lack of scientific support combined with the controversial nature of this classification would seem to indicate that it should not be included, or at a minimum, delayed for further evaluation.' (as quoted in De Angelis 1993:32)

Members of N.O.W. led a formal protest at the 1993 Annual Meeting of the American Psychiatric Association. Caplan and her associates put together a six-page statement for members of the APA (Committee for a Scientific and Responsible DSM 1993, "Before you vote on the DSM-IV Proposal about Premenstrual Syndrome, please read this"). The text of this position statement is contained in full in Caplan's book, so I will not go into details. However, the statement read in part like the statement put together in 1985 by the Coalition Against Misdiagnosis. One big difference was the emphasis on the legal implications of including PMDD in the DSM-IV. This statement read:

> Judicial decisions like those in the Dalkon Shield and the Meme breast implant cases make it absolutely clear that both individual physicians and groups that endorse particular actions (such as assignment of diagnostic categories) can be held liable for harm *especially when the research does not justify the action*. This is the case for placing 'Premenstrual Dysphoric Disorder' (PMDD) in the DSM-IV. (as found in Caplan 1985:148–149)

This and other interesting "insider" accounts of the DSM-IV process are contained in Caplan's recent book *They Say You're Crazy: How the World's Most Powerful Psychiatrists Decide Who's Normal* (1995). It contains Caplan's last attempt to prevent the APA from having the final word on the controversy since the DSM-IV is now published and widely used. In one interesting episode of what she calls "PMSgate," Caplan documents a case of what she calls "espionage" engaged in by a "mole" (one of Allen Frances' nephews) to uncover what was in her personal files about the DSM-IV (see Caplan 1995:131–133).

DSM-IV AND POLITICS AS USUAL

The events and actions that occurred during the DSM-IV controversy should not be surprising to those who have read this book and account of the DSM-III-R controversy. The professional, gendered, and scientific issues that helped to construct LLPDD continued, for the most part, to construct PMDD in the DSM-IV. Most accounts of the DSM-IV agreed that PMDD was the most contentious and publicized diagnosis (Seligmann 1993; De Angelis 1993; Solomon 1993; Vines 1994). For example: "A few categories in the new 900-page book have drawn criticism, especially the decision to classify a severe form of premenstrual syndrome called premenstrual dysphoric disorder (PMDD) as a mental illness in the appendix" (Squires 1994:10). And another account states the public reaction by Allen Frances:

> Though he tried to keep controversy to a minimum, clashes did occur over Self-Defeating Personality Disorder and Premenstrual Dysphoric Disorder.

Frances calls them 'tempests in a thimble' and laments that the media have overplayed the controversy by choosing to focus on these disorders. (Japenga 1994:20)

But the question remains: Why was the strategy/campaign not as effective as the one in 1985? The campaign to eliminate PMS/PMDD from the DSM-IV lost on all accounts. PMDD was located in the main text of the DSM-IV under the heading of a codable depression category (in spite of the evidence that PMDD was not just a depression). But why?

First, as the leader of the opposition forces, Paula Caplan did not have all the "requirements" to effectively fight within the APA. She is not a psychiatrist nor is she a PMS researcher. Thus, her arguments about the "bad science" involved in the PMS study evaluation were not seen as legitimate and thus were not as effective. On the other hand, neither did APA leaders listen to PMS expert and PMDD Advisory Member Sally Severino, who had major qualms about the scientific merit of including PMDD in the main text, especially as a depressive disorder. In a published debate about the arguments against including PMDD, PMS expert Mary Parlee framed this issue in professional politics:

Nothing in psychiatrists' professional norms or training or in the economic or social incentives of their jobs renders an argument in the form 'you [collectively] should not harm women [collectively]' particularly persuasive to them on either moral or practical grounds. (Parlee 1992:106)

She also indicated that Caplan and her co-authors are making a correct but ineffective argument about the "science" of PMDD:

In most cases it simply does not work—affect actual scientific practices—for feminists to critique research for not being in accord with verbally espoused and widely agreed-upon standards of rigorous scientific methodology. Research never is. What counts is whether the critique must be taken as sufficiently relevant by the researcher to require a defensive response, and that is determined by the positions and relative resources available to the researcher and critic. (Parlee 1992:106)

Parlee's point can be seen in pubic statements by Gold and Frances that indicate that they know the "stigmatization" argument, but that it did not sway them:

`Of course women still face discrimination and prejudice,' she [Gold] says, 'but you can't view every scientific study that has to do only with women as an offense against women. If we can say only a tiny group of women is ill, and they meet these specific criteria and can be helped, that's a *service* to women.' (as quoted in Solomon 1993:32)

For Frances, the public reason for including PMDD were as follows:

The reasons we included it were to stimulate research and to let women who have it know that it is a recognized problem they can get help for,' Dr. Frances said. 'The downside is that it might be stigmatizing to women.' (as quoted in Goleman 1994:C11)

The issue of stigmatization did not play as effectively in the controversy over DSM-IV for a variety of reasons. The first has something to do with introduction of antidepressant prescriptions for women's PMS by practicing psychiatrists. One of the stronger antiinclusion points against including LLPDD in the DSM-III-R controversy was that there was no effective treatment for this proposed diagnosis so there was no reason to differentially diagnose it from PMS. However, as discussed earlier, the rise of new medications such as Prozac and Xanax for the treatment of mood and, especially, depressive disorders had a major effect on the DSM-IV debate. Women have requested these new medications and physicians (especially psychiatrists) are prescribing them. However, the effective use of an antidepressant for the treatment of a purely physical disorder (PMS) is medically inconsistent. The medical solution to this seeming dilemma was the placement of PMDD in the main text of DSM-IV with a code number that also allows for the possibility of third-party insurance reimbursement of this newly declared psychiatric disorder. Since the cost of these new pharmaceutical products is expensive, women with insurance seem to have welcomed the inclusion of PMDD in the DSM-IV. This notion is supported, for example, in the following statement published by two psychiatrists in the introduction to their book:

Premenstrual syndrome and/or late luteal phase dysphoric disorder (proposed in the upcoming DSM-IV as depressive disorder not otherwise specified) are being contested as diagnostic entities by some feminists who are fearful of the scapegoating of women. Yet we have seen these disorders, and we must treat them both medically and psychiatrically if indicated. If premenstrual syndrome is not a psychiatric diagnosis, patients who could feel better with psychodynamic therapy or psychotropic medication will not have insurance coverage for treatment. (Bernstein and Lenhart 1992:xiv)

Note that once again the ubiquitous "feminists" returned in the DSM-IV debate. But now it is "some feminists" who are seen as blocking purported medical advances and the effective treatment of women, not to mention their economic well being. Proponents of the diagnosis become the more realistic supporters of women and their position in society:

> Proponents claim that the more specific designation would have several benefits. For one, they say, women suffering from PMDD won't be as likely to be condescendingly dismissed by physicians they consult. If they receive treatment for their symptoms, they'll have a better chance of reimbursement by insurance companies. (Seligmann 1993:66)

The new pharmaceutical treatment regimen is even being used on young girls with PMS. In an article about teenagers and PMS (where Jean Endicott is the "scientific expert" for the diagnosis and treatment of young girls for their PMS), the author indicates drug preferences:

> If she has severe emotional symptoms, many studies suggest she might be helped by antidepressants, such as Prozac, or a premenstrual dose of the antianxiety drug Xanax. In extreme cases, doctors may even put a girl's menstrual cycles on hold with a hormonal treatment such as danazol. (Debrovner 1993:54)

The rise of these new drugs and the subsequent use by both women and young girls helped to both complicate and simplify the issues in the DSM-IV controversy. The effective treatment of these drugs complicated the arguments against the inclusion of PMDD in the DSM-IV and simplified the arguments for its inclusion.

Another reason why I believe that the opposition forces were not as effective in the DSM-IV controversy is that PMDD stood alone to the charge that it was stigmatizing to women. In the DSM-III-R controversy, Paraphilic Rapism and Masochistic Personality Disorder (later named Self-Defeating Personality Disorder) were grouped together with LLPDD as potential diagnoses that were stigmatizing to all women. This tactic brought together women's groups and mental health professionals with diverse interests and concerns in fighting the inclusion of all of these diagnoses in the DSM-III-R. This connection to other so-called misogynistic diagnoses was lost early in the DSM-IV process when Self-Defeating Personality Disorder was removed from further consideration (Holden 1993). And, consistent with the tactic of claiming that the DSM-IV was "scientifically based," it was removed for lack of evidence. Science was portrayed as winning out over the professional interests of psychoanalysts and the political claims of feminists. And as a result, PMDD stood alone in being portrayed as the diagnosis that was potentially harmful to women (see Caplan 1995).

I also believe that Caplan's threatened lawsuit was very negatively perceived by psychiatrists and the APA and that this may have affected some of her credibility. For example, Lehman portrays the issue in the following account:

> Caplan is so incensed about the decision that she has written to members of the American Psychiatric Association's voting assembly threatening to sue them if they vote for or use the diagnosis, saying that it will harm women just as defective medical devices do. (Lehman 1993:36)

In response to this threat, Lehman indicates that

> Two leading Boston psychiatrists, Dr. Malkah Notman and Dr. Carol Nadelson, say they see strengths in the arguments on both sides, that the debate raises real issues that cannot easily be reconciled. Both said, however, they thought threatening psychiatrists with lawsuits is not a constructive strategy. (Lehman 1993:36)

In 1986, the threatened lawsuit by Lenore Walker about the inclusion of Self-Defeating Personality Disorder in the DSM-III-R never materialized. Why would the APA and its leaders take another threatened lawsuit seriously? It was a threat that was not taken seriously but did seem to annoy APA leaders.

Finally, the major difference between the controversy over LLPDD and PMDD has to do with a term that I now call "Identity Science." Identity Science involves the personal identification of a scientist with the research topic when it is being debated or contested. For example, when Simon Levay first published his research on the "Gay Brain," much was made of the fact that Levay was a gay man. Ironically, instead of detracting from LeVay's scientific claims, his "Gayness" has tended to lend further support and credence to his study. If LeVay is gay and his science and scientific credentials are good, then the research must be true. For example, the following account was found in *Nature*:

> But, of course, there is no reason why a result that is surprising should be scorned on that account alone, while those who know LeVay attest to the excellence of his work in neuroanatomy. (LeVay also volunteers that he is himself a homosexual.) So skepticism is inappropriate. (Maddox 1991:13)

Thus, identity science goes beyond just personal identification with the individual scientist. It is used as a political measures to justify a controversial area of research. People who shares the personal characteristics of the group under study would not willingly subject themselves to potential negative consequences of that research. This seems logical and reasonable to most people, which is why it is a subtle political process.

In the LLPDD controversy, the anti-inclusion scientists (such as Hamilton and Alagna) used their personal identification as feminists to suggest that LLPDD stigmatized all women. Proinclusion scientists relied only on their credentials as scientists to argue that LLPDD was not stigmatizing. Therefore, press accounts and many psychiatrists portrayed the debate (as suggested in Chapter 6) as a battle between scientists and feminists and discounted many of the "feminist" arguments against the inclusion of LLPDD.

The DSM-IV debate about PMDD signified a significant change in this public portrayal and identification of the "feminist." The APA first appointed an all-women PMDD work group (the members are discussed earlier in this chapter). The point that this group was composed of all women was frequently pointed out in discussions of the diagnosis:

> Stressing that PMS is not a mental disorder, the American Psychiatric Association assembled an all-woman work group to evaluate what in the appendix of *DSM-IIIR* is called late luteal phase dysphoric disorder. (Cotton 1993:14)

How could an all-women work group work against all women by voting to include a stigmatizing disorder? But having an all-women work group was not the only way that identity science was used differently in the PMDD controversy. After all, the majority of the LLPDD work group were women, and they still voted to include LLPDD in the DSM-III-R (see Chapter 3) and although this was referred to in the DSM-III-R controversy, not as much was made of it by APA leaders.

The issue in the DSM-IV revisions was not just that this was an area of dispute that *women* could disagree upon, but that now even *"feminists"* could disagree over it. Between 1987 and 1994, the work group members took on the public label of "feminist" to go with their identity as "women." For example, the following statement was made during the controversy by one of its members: "'Every one of the women in the group counts herself a feminist and felt a strong responsibility to do the best she could for women, but saw that in the end as something different,' says Frank" (as quoted in Span 1993:C2). Jean Endicott also declared herself as a public feminist in the DSM-IV debate: "Dr. Endicott said she considers herself a feminist and agrees in spirit with some of the sociocultural concerns expressed by feminist psychologists. But she sees the issues somewhat differently, she said" (De Angelis 1993:33). By taking on the public label of "feminist," consciously or not, the all-women PMDD work group was able to deflect controversy away from the possible stigmatizing effects of the diagnosis. By deflecting these concerns as a broader cultural issue of stigmatizing all people with mental illness and away from the APA specifically stigmatizing just women, the public debate about this scientific controversy was clouded and complicated—which resulted in less outcry about the inclusion of the diagnosis in the DSM-IV.

THE SETTLEMENT

When the dust settled and the DSM-IV was published, only minor changes were made to the existing criteria for Premenstrual Dysphoric Disorder (ordering and one addition to the symptom list) and the wording remained similar to that of Late Luteal Phase Dysphoric Disorder (American Psychiatric Association 1994:718–719). Interestingly, and maybe not so coincidentally, the symptom category "markedly depressed mood, feelings of hopelessness,, or self-deprecating thoughts" was moved from number 4 on the DSM-III-R list to number 1 on the DSM-IV list. This would correspond to the new emphasis on PMDD as a depressive disorder. An eleventh symptom category, "a subjective sense of being overwhelmed or out of control," was added to the previous 10 symptoms. Finally, the additional requirement of having at least two "consecutive" symptomatic cycles was added.

The theme that science and merit were shaping the DSM-IV rather than the personalities and loud voices of the DSM-III-R developers was played upon throughout DSM-IV development, and especially with its publication in 1994. For example, one writer stated: "Frances sought to avoid the controversies that divided previous DSM committees by placing less emphasis on input from the public and special interest groups" (Japenga 1994:20). In another article Frances stated: "But the biggest change in the manual is the way in which it was compiled, a six-year process that relied on empirical scientific data rather than on expert consensus" (as quoted in Squires 1994:10). Frances also claimed in another article, that "[t]here's been a stronger emphasis on research data than with previous revisions. That has made people less contentious. They couldn't argue just from ideology anymore" (as quoted in Goleman 1994:C1). Pincus, vice-chair of the Task Force, proclaimed (somewhat ironically): "This wasn't just a bunch of guys sitting around a table deciding what should be in DSM-IV" (as quoted in Squires 1994:10).

Even DSM critics agreed that Frances was able to avoid *substantial* controversy and did hold the line on the proliferation of new diagnoses. Kutchins and Kirk write:

> Allen Frances, who oversaw the compilation of D.S.M.-IV, has largely avoided controversy this time around. When he took over the revision task force, he announced that it would stress science over politics and personalities.

More than 1,000 experts, mainly psychiatrists, reviewed a mountain of scientific studies to guide their revisions, and higher standards were used to
evaluate more than 100 proposed new diagnoses. Unlike prior revisions that
included new diagnoses even when the scientific support for them was
skimpy, the tightened standards permitted only eight new categories. (Kirk
and Kutchins 1994:17)

However, in DSM-IV, the psychiatric profession answered its critics in a
manner similar to the DSM-III-R settlement; they ultimately tried to daz-
zle us with "Science" by continually stressing the "scientific merits" of
DSM-IV. This was a conscious professional strategy similar to the settlement of the controversy over LLPDD discussed in Chapter 7 and to what
Kirk and Kutchins (1992) describe in their book *The Selling of DSM*. The
"empirical" development of DSM-IV was consciously contrasted rhetori-
cally to the "political" decisions made in DSM-III and DSM-III-R. This was
done in part by answering charges of its critics "regarding the scientific basis of DSM-III and DSM-III-R that noted the lack of systematic review or
documentation of the decisions made in these editions" (Frances et al.
1994:209). For example, Frances often made that claim that"More than any
other nomenclature of mental disorders, DSM-IV . . . is grounded in empirical evidence" (as quoted in Cotton 1993:13).

The APA was publicly "holding the line of proliferation of new diagnoses." Perhaps more importantly it was revisiting professional boundary
disputes within psychiatry, with other mental health professions, as well
as reaffirming its relationship to the medical profession. In the DSM-IV, the
authors consciously blurred the distinctions of "Organic" versus "Inor-
ganic" Disorders and "Mental" versus "Medical" Conditions." A journalist reports this change: "Also reclassified is a whole section on diseases
dubbed 'organic' in the previous DSM edition. They are now peppered
throughout the new DSM-IV, and identified as being due to a general
medical condition" (Squires 1994:10). An article in *Journal of the American
Medical Association* also documents this shift: "The terms 'organic' and
'nonorganic' diseases have been eliminated on the grounds that they imply a mind/body dualism and that some mental disorders are not true
medical illnesses" (Cotton 1993:13). The author describes this blending as
a result of a "shift away from psychoanalytic conceptions toward an approach based more in biology" (Cotton 1993:13).

Robert Spitzer is also quoted in this article as saying: "We certainly all
believe that for major mental disorders there is something biologically not
right." And, he says, "it stigmatizes the patient because it suggests that primary psychiatric disorders are not really medical disorders" (as quoted in
Cotton 1993:13). This notion that psychiatric disorders are "medical disorders" is an important statement, as psychiatry continued its emphasis on

the profession as a medical profession. This controversy started with the debate over Spitzer and Endicott's statement in the DSM-III and DSM-III-R debate that "mental disorders are a subset of medical disorders" (see Chapter 5 for a discussion of this point). With the publication of DSM-IV, Spitzer's perspective on this point was finally validated in the DSM (and as official APA policy).

At the same time, the APA was "mindful" of its sometimes tenuous relationship to other mental health and health associations. As stated in Chapter 5, the APA reached out to other organizations in the DSM-IV revision process and tried to inform them about what was happening. The American Psychiatric Association was able to effectively bring other professional groups into the process of constructing DSM-IV. The leaders of the APA reached out and created formal liaisons to other professional groups for the revisions of DSM-IV. In an effective way in the DSM-IV revision process, the APA leaders were able to enroll their critics as allies to reduce dissent and public controversy (see Latour 1987 for the complete discussion of this process). The APA and DSM-IV leadership effectively also brought in Consumer Groups such as the National Alliance for the Mentally Ill to argue that the debate over DSM-IV consisted of the broader issue of stigmatizing people with mental illness and the controversy over PMDD could be framed as a general issue of stigmatization and not just a gender stigmatizing issue.

ANOTHER BLACK BOX BUT THE QUESTIONS REMAIN THE SAME

PMDD and the DSM-IV have now been black boxed but not without considerable (and as I have shown) unwanted public attention once again being given to the social and political nature of the DSM and its revisions. What I have tried to document in the study of a PMS-related diagnosis in both the DSM-III-R and the DSM-IV is that no matter how scientists and psychiatrists try to portray the development of the DSM, all science is political. What is especially aggravating is that the developers of the DSM-IV want the public to be swayed by the "empirical" and "nonpolitical" nature of DSM-IV. No products of culture—even ones with the label of "empirical" and "scientifically based"—are free from the social, political, and even economic considerations of their human creators.

One of the Task Force members comes to this conclusion in his assessment of the DSM-IV and the controversy over PMDD. Peter Nathan is a psychologist who was also a member of the DSM-IV Task Force and of the Substance Use Disorders Work Group:

the fact remains that when empirical data that would justify a deciiion are judged to be unavailable and a decision nonetheless is required, one of the bases for such a decision by successive Task Forces has been prevailing political sentiment. By itself neither good nor bad, it is nonetheless true that basing an important decision about a diagnosis on political sentiment when the rhetoric has been that it is empirical findings that have guided these decisions is misleading at best, dishonest at worst. (Nathan 1994:108)

I could not have said it better myself. Science is politics, but when scientists try to hide behind the mask and authority of science, it is up to us to challenge this assumption. To think otherwise is to be fooled by science. No one wants to be a fool. The case of LLPDD in the DSM-III-R and PMDD in the DSM-IV cannot be accounted for by single explanations. There are similarities to the events and professional, gendered, and scientific meanings and strategies that people gave to these diagnostic categories, but there were also major differences in terms of the structural conditions and actors in the development of the DSM-III-R and DSM-IV. In addition, multiple interests and actors were involved in both controversies. This book has asked you to consider scientific controversies as consisting of multiple arenas of action and opinion in which there are no easy or simple explanations.

NOTES

1.   I did not engage in the same in-depth analysis of records and interviews in my study of the DSM-IV controversy. My analysis is based upon documents that have been made public in publication [e.g., the recent book by Caplan (1995) and the DSM-IV itself] or statements made and published in the press and the interviews I conducted for the DSM-III-R controversy.

2.   As we see in this chapter, Spitzer may have not been "in charge," but found a way to keep involved through interviews with newspapers and journals about the development of the DSM-IV.

3.   Frances is currently the Chair of the Psychiatry Department at Duke University.

4.   Not all of the press accounts portray Stotland's position as totally against the inclusion of PMDD in the DSM-IV [e.g., see the article by Chase (1993) in the *Wall Street Journal*]. Stotland's lack of consistency and clarity about an antiinclusion position is explored by Caplan (1995).

5.   In fact, in my own research writings on this subject I was encouraged and in one particular case told to use a header "research criteria" instead of diagnostic criteria in numerous communications with the American Psychiatric Association Press. In this book, I have not chosen to use their language for the following reasons. I do not believe that it is accurate. The criteria are *not* just being used for re-

search purposes. Women were being given the diagnosis of Late Luteal Phase Dysphoric Disorder and are now given the diagnosis of Premenstrual Dysphoric Disorder from the criteria set out in the DSM-III-R and the DSM-IV.

6.   In one study, "37 percent of the women taking Xanax described a 50 percent improvement in their daily symptoms from descriptions taken before treatment, compared with 29 percent in the progesterone group and 30 percent in the placebo group" (quoted in Donnelly 1995:12A). This is worrisome, since there is only a 7% difference between Xanax and a placebo and since Xanax is a habit-forming drug. The authors of the study recognize this and recommend a limited dose of the drug to the luteal phase. Yet the luteal phase can consist of 2 out of every 4 weeks (see Freeman et al., 1995). The Prozac study indicated a better success with a lower dosage (20 versus 60 mg a day) than the placebo, but could not state whether a woman should stay on Prozac all the time or whether a single dose in the premenstrual phase is just as efficacious (see Steiner et al., 1995).

7.   Neither Caplan nor I am really sure what the difference between a consultant and an adviser is (see Caplan 1995:11).

References

Abbott, Andrew. 1988. *The System of Professions: An Essay of the Division of Expert Labor.* Chicago: University of Chicago Press.

Abplanalp, Judith. 1983. "Premenstrual Syndrome: A Selective Review." *Women & Health* 8(2–3):107–123.

Adler, Tina. 1990a. "Causes, Cure of PMS Still Elude Researchers." *APA Monitor* January:10.

———. 1990b. "PMS Diagnosis Draws Fire from Researchers." *APA Monitor* January:12.

Allen, Hilary. 1990. "At the Mercy of Her Hormones: Premenstrual Tension and the Law." Pp. 200–228 in *The Woman in Question*, edited by Parveen Adams and Elizabeth Cowie. Cambridge MA: The MIT Press.

American Psychiatric Association. 1952. *Diagnostic and Statistical Manual of Mental Disorders.* Washington, DC: The American Psychiatric Association.

———. 1968. *Diagnostic and Statistical Manual of Mental Disorders*, Second Edition. Washington, DC: The American Psychiatric Association.

———. 1980. *Diagnostic and Statistical Manual of Mental Disorders*, Third Edition. Washington, DC: The American Psychiatric Association.

———. 1987. *Diagnostic and Statistical Manual of Mental Disorders*, Third Edition, Revised. Washington, DC: The American Psychiatric Association.

———. 1994. *Diagnostic and Statistical Manual of Mental Disorders*, Fourth Edition. Washington, DC: American Psychiatric Association Press.

Barnes, Barry. 1977. *Interests and the Growth of Knowledge.* London: Routledge and Kegan Paul.

Barton, Walter. 1987. *The History and Influence of the American Psychiatric Association.* Washington, DC: American Psychiatric Association Press.

Baxter, William, and David Hathcox III. 1994. *America's Care of The Mentally Ill: A Photographic History.* Washington, DC: American Psychiatric Press.

Bayer, Ronald. 1987. *Homosexuality and American Psychiatry: The Politics of Diagnosis.* Princeton, NJ: Princeton University Press.

Becker, Howard. 1982. *Art Worlds.* Chicago: University of Chicago Press.

Bell, Susan. 1986. "Premenstrual Syndrome and the Medicalization of Menopause: A Sociological Perspective." Pp. 151–174 in *Premenstrual Syndrome*, edited by Benson Ginsburg and Bonnie F. Carter. New York: Plenum Press.

———. 1987. "Changing Ideas: The Medicalization of Menopause." *Social Science and Medicine* 24:535–542.

Bender, Stephanie. 1989. *PMS Questions and Answers.* Los Angeles: The Body Press.

Benedek, Elissa. 1988. "Premenstrual Syndrome: A View from the Bench." *Journal of Clinical Psychiatry* 49(12):498–502.

Berlant, Jeffrey. 1974. *Professions and Monopoly: A Study of Medicine in the United States and Great Britain.* Los Angeles: University of California Press.

Bernstein, Anne E., and Sharyn A. Lenhart. 1992. *The Psychodynamic Treatment of Women.* Washington, DC: American Psychiatric Press.

Bevins, George. 1990. *"Creationism, Fraud, the New Age and Animal Rights: Opening and Closure in Scientific Controversies."* Indiana University, unpublished manuscript.

Bijker, Wiebe, Thomas Hughes, and Trevor Pinch (eds). 1987. *The Social Construction of Technological Systems.* Cambridge, MA: MIT Press.

Blashfield, Roger. 1984. *The Classification of Psychopathology: Neo-Kraepelinian and Quantitative Approaches.* New York: Plenum Press.

Bloor, David. 1981. "The Strengths of the Strong Programme." *Philosophy of the Social Sciences* 11:199–213.

Blume, Elizabeth. 1983. "Methodological Difficulties Plague PMS Research." *Journal of the American Medical Association* 249:2866.

Blumenthal, Susan, and Carol Nadelson. 1988. "Late Luteal Phase Dysphoric Disorder (Premenstrual Syndromes): Clinical Implications." *Journal of Clinical Psychiatry* 49(12):469–474.

Boston Women's Health Collective. 1973. *Our Bodies, Ourselves.* New York: Simon & Schuster.

———. 1992a. *The New Our Bodies, Ourselves: Updated and Expanded for the '90s.* New York: Simon & Schuster.

———. 1992b. "How Real is PMS?" *Ms.* II(4):75–76.

Boxer, Sarah. 1987. "The Parable of the Cheek-Turners and the Cheek-Smiters." *Discover* (August):80–83.

Broverman, K., Broverman, D. M., Clarkson, F. E., Rosenkrantz, P. S. and Vogel, S. R. 1970. "Sex Role Stereotypes and Clinical Judgement of Mental Health." *Journal of Consulting and Clinical Psychology* 34:1–7.

Brown, E. Richard. 1979. *Rockefeller Medicine Men: Medicine and Capitalism in America.* Berkeley: University of California Press.

Brown, Laura. 1985. "Masochistic Personality Disorder Rears Its Ugly Head." *FTI Interchange* 3(3):1–2.

Brown, Phil. 1987. "Diagnostic Conflict and Contradiction in Psychiatry." *Journal of Health and Social Behavior* 27 (March):37–50.

———. 1990. "The Name Game: Toward a Sociology of Diagnosis." *The Journal of Mind and Behavior* 11(3 & 4):385–406.

Bucher, Rue. 1966. "Pathology: A Study of Social Movements Within a Profession." Pp. 113–127 in *Medical Men and Their Work*, edited by Eliot Freidson and Judith Lorber. Chicago: Aldine.

Bucher, Rue, and Anselm Strauss. 1961. "Professions in Process." *American Journal of Sociology* 66:325–334.

Buckley, Thomas, and Alma Gottlieb. 1988. *Blood Magic: The Anthropology of Menstruation.* Berkeley: University of California Press.

Callon, Michel. 1987. "Society in the Making: The Study of Technology as a Tool for Sociological Analysis." Pp. 83–106 in *The Social Construction of Technological Systems*, edited by Wiebe Bijker, Thomas Hughes, and Trevor Pinch. Cambridge, MA: MIT Press.

Caplan, Paula. 1985. *The Myth of Women's Masochism*, 1st edition. New York: Dutton.

———. 1991. "How Do They Decide Who Is Normal? The Bizarre, But True, Tale of the DSM Process." *Canadian Psychology* 32(2):162–170.

———. 1992."Gender Issues in the Diagnosis of Mental Disorder." *Women & Therapy* 12(4):71–82.

———. 1995. *They Say You're Crazy: How the World's Most Powerful Psychiatrists Decide Who's Normal*. Reading, MA: Addison-Wesley.

Caplan, Paula, Joan McCurdy-Myers, and Maureen Gans. 1992. "Should 'Premenstrual Syndrome' Be Called a Psychiatric Abnormality?" *Feminism & Psychology* 2(1):27–44.

Carey, Joseph. 1986. "Is PMS Mental Illness? Debate Grows." *U.S. News & World Report* 100(May 26):60.

Carr-Saunders, A. M., and P. A. Wilson. 1933. *The Professions*. Oxford: Clarendon.

Chaite, Linda. 1986. "Premenstrual Syndrome and Our Sisters in Crime: A Feminist Dilemma." *Women's Rights Law Reporter* 9(3–4):267–293

Chase, Marilyn. 1993. "Version of PMS Called Disorder by Psychiatrists." *Wall Street Journal*, May 28, B1, B3.

Chesler, Phyllis. [1972] 1989. *Women and Madness*. San Diego: Harcourt, Brace Jovanovich.

Chodoff, Paul. 1986. "DSM-III and Psychotherapy." *American Journal of Psychiatry* 143(2):201–203.

Chrisler, Joan, and Karen Levy. 1990. "The Media Construct a Menstrual Monster: A Content Analysis of PMS Articles in the Popular Press." *Women & Health* 16(2):89–104.

Clarke, Adele. 1990a. "Women's Health: Life-Cycle Issues." Pp. 3–40 in *Women, Health and Medicine in America: A Historical Handbook*, edited by Rima D. Apple. New York: Garland.

———. 1990b. "A Social Worlds Research Adventure: The Case of Reproductive Science." Pp. 15–42 in *Theories of Science in Society*, edited by Susan Cozzens and Thomas Gieryn. Bloomington, IN: Indiana University Press.

Clarke, Adele, and Theresa Montini. 1993. "The Many Faces of RU486: Tales of Situated Knowledges and Technological Contestations." *Science, Technology & Human Values* 18(1):42–78.

Cogan, Morris. 1953. "Toward a Definition of a Profession." *Harvard Educational Review* 23 (Winter):33–50.

Conrad, Peter, and Joseph Schneider. 1980. *Deviance and Medicalization: From Badness to Sickness*. St. Louis: C. V. Mosby.

Corea, Gena. [1975] 1985. *The Hidden Malpractice: How American Medicine Mistreats Women*, Updated Edition. New York: Harper Colophon Books.

Cotton, Paul. 1993. "Psychiatrists Set to Approve DSM-IV." *Journal of the American Medical Association* 270(1):13–15.

Daily Bulletin of the 139th Annual Meeting of the American Psychiatric Association. 1986a. *DSM Symposium to Air Three Issues*. Third Issue, Tuesday, May 13th:1–2.

———. 1986b. *AWP Opposes DSM Shifts*. Third Issue, Tuesday, May 13th:2.

Dalton, Katharina. [1979] 1983. *Once A Month*. Claremont, CA: Hunter House.

Dan, Alice, and Linda Lewis. 1992. *Menstrual Health in Women's Lives*. Urbana: University of Illinois Press.

De Angelis, Tori. 1993. "Controversial Diagnosis Is Voted into Latest DSM: Opponents Cite Potential of Harm to Women." *APA Monitor* (September):32–33.

Debrovner, Diane. 1993. "PMS: Not Just for Grownups: Misdiagnosing Girlish Moodiness Can Have Tragic Results." *Longevity* June:54.

Delaney, Janice, Mary Lupton, and Emily Toth. 1988. *The Curse: A Cultural History of Menstruation*. Chicago: University of Illinois Press.

DePaul, Amy. 1986. "Defining New Diseases of the Mind: Feminist Groups Complain That a Diagnosis of PMS Will Cause Discrimination." *Washington Post* March 5 (Health Section):20.

Dire, Angela. 1986. "NOW Assails Proposal of Psychiatrists." *Rocky Mountain News* June 14, 1986.

Donnelly, Kathleen. 1995. "Experts rule out Prozac, Xanax as PMS Cure-alls." *San Jose Mercury News* July 16:1A, 12A.

Eagan, Andrea. 1983. "The Selling of Premenstrual Syndrome: Who Profits from Making PMS 'The Disease of the 80s'?" *Ms.* October:26–31.

Ehrenreich, Barbara, and Deidre English. 1973a. *Complaints and Disorders: The Sexual Politics of Sickness*. Old Westbury, NY: Feminist Press.

Ehrenreich, Barbara, and Deidre English. 1973b. *Witches, Midwives and Nurses: A History of Women Healers*. Old Westbury, NY: Feminist Press.

Ehrenreich, Barbara, and Deidre English. 1978. *For Her Own Good: 150 Years of the Experts' Advice to Women*. Garden City, NY: Anchor Press/Doubleday.

Ehrlich, Frederick. 1985. "OTCs: All Eyes on Ibuprofen While PMS Product Sales Soar." *Drug Topics* 129 (July 1):45–55.

Encyclopedia of Associations. 1985. Edited by M. Fisk. MI: Gale Research Company.

———. 1989. Edited by M. Fisk. MI: Gale Research Company.

———. 1991. Edited by M. Fisk. MI: Gale Research Company.

Erickson, Kai. 1966. *Wayward Puritans: A Study in the Sociology of Deviance*. New York: John Wiley.

Fausto-Sterling, Anne. 1985. *Myths of Gender: Biological Theories about Women and Men*. New York: Basic Books.

Fee, Elizabeth (ed.). 1983. *Women and Health: The Politics of Sex in Medicine*. Farmingdale, NY: Baywood Publishing Company.

Fleck, Ludwig. [1935] 1977. *Genesis and Development of a Scientific Fact*. Chicago: University of Chicago Press.

Figert, Anne. 1995. "The Three Faces of PMS: The Professional, Gendered, and Scientific Structuring of a Psychiatric Disorder." *Social Problems* 42(1):56–73.

Fink, Paul. 1987. "Foreword" to Ginsburg, Benson, and Bonnie F. Carter (eds.), *Premenstrual Syndrome: Ethical and Legal Implications in a Biomedical Perspective*. New York: Plenum Press.

Fisher, Kathleen. 1986a. "DSM-III-R Amendment Process Frustrates Non-MD's." *APA Monitor* February:17–24.

———. 1986b. "DSM-III-R Protest: Critics Say Psychiatry Has Been Stonewalling." *APA Monitor* July:4–5.

Fox, Renee. 1977. "The Medicalization and Demedicalization of American Society." *Daedalus* 106:9–22.

Frances, Allen, Thomas Widiger, and Harold Pincus. 1989. "The Development of DSM-IV." *Archives of General Psychiatry* 46:373–375.

Frances, Allen, Harold Pincus, Thomas Widiger, Wendy Davis, and Michael First. 1990. "DSM-IV: Work in Progress." *American Journal of Psychiatry* 147(11):1439–1448.

Frances, Allen, Michael First, Thomas Widiger, Gloria Miele, Sarah Tilly, Wendy Davis, and Harold Pincus. 1991. "An A to Z Guide to DSM-IV Conundrums." *Journal of Abnormal Psychology* 100:407–412.

Frances, Allen, Avram Mack, Michael First, Thomas Widiger, Ruth Ross, Leslie Forman, and Wendy Davis. 1994. "DSM-IV Meets Philosophy." *The Journal of Medicine and Philosophy* 19:207–218.

Frank, Robert. 1931. "The Hormonal Causes of Premenstrual Tension." *Archives of Neurology and Psychiatry* 26:1053–1057.

Freeman, Ellen, Karl Rickels, Steven Sondheimer, and Marcia Polansky. 1995. "A Double-blind Trial of Oral Progesterone, Alprazolam, and Placebo in Treatment of Severe Premenstrual Syndrome." *Journal of the American Medical Association* 274(1):51–57.

Freidson, Eliot. 1970a. *Professional Dominance*. New York: Atherton Press.

———. 1970b. *The Profession of Medicine*. New York: Dodd, Mead.

———. 1986. *Professional Powers: A Study of the Institutionalization of Formal Knowledge*. Chicago: University of Chicago Press.

Fujimura, Joan. 1988. "Constructing Doable Problems in Cancer Research: Where Social Worlds Meet." *Social Problems* 35:261–283.

Gaines, Atwood. 1992. "From DSM-I to III-R; Voices of Self, Mastery and the Other: A Cultural Constructivist Reading of U.S. Psychiatric Classification." *Social Science and Medicine* 35(1):3–24.

Gieryn, Thomas F. 1983. "Boundary-Work and the Demarcation of Science from Non-Science: Strains and Interests in Professional Ideologies of Scientists." *American Sociological Review* 48:781–795.

———. 1994. "Boundaries of Science." Pp. 393–443 in *Handbook of Science, Technology and Society*, edited by S. Jasanoff, G. Markle, J. Petersen, and T. Pinch. Beverly Hills, CA: Sage.

Gieryn, Thomas, and Anne Figert. 1986. "Scientists Protect Their Cognitive Authority: The Status Degradation Ceremony of Sir Cyril Burt." In *The Sociology of the Sciences Yearbook* (The Knowledge Society), Volume X, edited by G. Bohme and N. Stehr. Dordrecht: D. Reidel.

Gieryn, Thomas, and Anne Figert. 1990. "Ingredients for a Theory of Science in Society: O-Rings, Ice Water, C-Clamp, Richard Feynman and the Press." Pp. 67–97 in *Theories of Science in Society*, edited by Susan Cozzens and Thomas Gieryn. Bloomington, IN: Indiana University Press

Gieryn, Thomas, George Bevins, and Stephen Zehr. 1985. "Professionalization of American Scientists: Public Science and the Creation/Evolution Trials." *American Sociological Review* 50:392–409.

Gilbert, G. Nigel, and Michael Mulkay. 1984. *Opening Pandora's Box: A Sociological Analysis of Scientists' Discourse*. Cambridge: Cambridge University Press.

Ginsburg, Benson, and Bonnie F. Carter (eds.). 1986. *Premenstrual Syndrome: Ethical and Legal Implications in a Biomedical Perspective*. New York: Plenum Press.

Gitlin, Michael, and Robert Pasnau. 1989. "Psychiatric Syndromes Linked to Reproductive Function in Women: A Review of Current Knowledge." *American Journal of Psychiatry* 146:1413–1422.

Gold, Judith. 1994. "Historical Perspective of Premenstrual Syndrome." Pp. 171–183 in *Premenstrual Dysphorias: Myths and Realities*, edited by Judith Gold and Sally Severino. Washington, DC: American Psychiatric Press.

Gold, Judith, and Sally Severino. 1994. *Premenstrual Dysphorias: Myths and Realities.* Washington, DC: American Psychiatric Press.

Goleman, Daniel. 1985. "New Psychiatric Syndromes Spur Protest." *The New York Times* November 19, 1985:C1,C16.

———. 1994."Revamping Psychiatrists' Bible." *The New York Times* April 19, 1994:C1,C11.

Golub, Sharon. 1992. *Periods: From Menarche to Menopause.* Newbury Park, CA: Sage.

Goode, William. 1957. "Community within a Community: The Professions." *American Sociological Review* 22:194–200.

Goodman, Ellen. 1986. "Cursed and Pre-Cursed." *The Washington Post*, May 24:A25.

Goodwin, Donald, and Samuel Guze. 1989. Preface to Donald Goodwin and Samuel Guze, *Psychiatric Diagnosis*, fourth edition. New York: Oxford University Press.

Gottlieb, Alma. 1988. "American Premenstrual Syndrome." *Anthropology Today* 4(6):10–13.

Gould, Stephen Jay. 1981. *The Mismeasure of Man.* New York: W. W. Norton.

Greene, Raymond, and Katharina Dalton. 1953. "The Premenstrual Syndrome." *British Medical Journal* 1:1007–1014.

Grob, Gerald. 1983. *Mental Illness and American Society*, 1875–1940. Princeton, NJ: Princeton University Press.

———. 1985. *The Inner World of American Psychiatry, 1890–1940.* New Brunswick, NJ: Rutgers University Press.

———. 1991. *From Asylum to Community.* Princeton, NJ: Princeton University Press.

———. 1994. *The Mad Among Us.* New York: The Free Press.

Gusfield, Joseph. 1989. "Constructing the Ownership of Social Problems: Fun and Profit in the Welfare State." *Social Problems* 36(5):431–441.

Guttentag, Marcia, Susan Salasin, and Deborah Belle (eds.). 1980. *The Mental Health of Women.* New York: Academic Press.

Hamilton, Jean. 1988. "Special Commentary: Is Media Coverage on the Diagnostic Controversy an Index of History in-the-Making for Women and Science?" *Coalition Report: Newsletter of the National Coalition for Women's Mental Health* Fall 1987/Spring 1988:9–11.

Hamilton, Jean, and Alagna, Sheryle. 1986. *Premenstrual Dysphoric Disorder.* Paper presented in the debate: "Controversies in the Revision of DSM-III." Annual meeting of the American Psychiatric Association, Washington, DC, May 1986.

Hamilton, Jean, and Gallant, Sheryle. 1988. "On a Premenstrual Diagnosis: What's in a Name?" *Professional Psychology: Research and Practice* 19(3):271–278.

Hamilton, Jean, and Gallant, Sheryle. 1990. "Problematic Aspects of Diagnosing

Premenstrual Phase Dysphoria: Recommendations for Psychological Research and Practice." *Professional Psychology: Research and Practice* 21(1):60–68.

Heneson, Nancy (with Celia Strain). 1984. "The Selling of P.M.S." *Science '84* 5(May):6671.

Holden, Constance. 1986. "Proposed New Psychiatric Diagnoses Raise Charges of Gender Bias." *Science* 231:327–328.

Holden, Constance. 1993. "Revising Psychiatric Diagnoses." *Science* 260:1586–1587.

Hood, Kathryn. 1992. "Contextual Determinants of Menstrual Cycle Effects in Observations of Social Interactions." Pp. 83–97 in *Menstrual Health in Women's Lives*, edited by Alice Dan and Linda Lewis. Urbana: University of Illinois Press.

Horney, Karen. [1931] 1967. "Premenstrual Tension." Pp. 99–106 in *Feminine Psychology*, edited by Harold Kelman. New York: Norton.

Hubbard, Ruth. 1990. *The Politics of Women's Biology*. New Brunswick, NJ: Rutgers University Press.

Hughes, Thomas. 1987. "The Evolution of Large Technological Systems." Pp. 51–82 in *The Social Construction of Technological Systems*, edited by Wiebe Bijker, Thomas Hughes, and Trevor Pinch. Cambridge, MA: MIT Press.

Institute for Research on Women's Health (IRWH). 1985. *Briefing Book on: A PMS-Related Psychiatric Diagnosis*. Unpublished manuscript.

Jacobus, Mary, Evelyn Fox Keller, and Sally Shuttleworth. 1990. *Body/Politics: Women and the Discourses of Science*. New York: Routledge.

Japenga, Ann. 1994. "Rewriting the Dictionary of Madness." *Los Angeles Times Magazine* June 5, 1994:18–20, 34–37.

Jasanoff, Sheila. 1987. "EPA's Regulation of Daminozide: Unscrambling the Messages of Risk." *Science, Technology & Human Values* 12(3 &4):116–124.

Johnson, Thomas. 1987. "Premenstrual Syndrome as a Western Culture Specific Disorder." *Culture, Medicine and Psychiatry* 11:337–356.

Kaplan, Marcie. 1983. "A Woman's View of DSM-III." *American Psychologist* 38:786–792.

Kass-Annese, Barbara, and Hal Danzer. 1987. *Say Good-Bye to PMS: The Step-By-Step Guide That Lets You Help Yourself!* New York: Warner Books.

Keye, William R. 1988. *The Premenstrual Syndrome*. Philadelphia: Saunders.

Keyser, Lucy. 1986. "APA Cuts Manual to Please Feminists." *The Washington Times* July 4:80.

Kirk, Stuart. 1986. "A Last Dance With Freud." *Newsweek* October 13:15.

Kirk, Stuart, and Herb Kutchins. 1992. *The Selling of DSM: The Rhetoric of Science in Psychiatry*. Hawthorne, NY: Aldine de Gruyter.

———. 1994. "Is Bad Writing a Mental Disorder?" *New York Times* June 20, Sec A:17.

Kirk, Stuart, Max Siporin, and Herb Kutchins. 1989. "The Prognosis for Social Work Diagnosis." *Social Casework: The Journal of Contemporary Social Work* 70:295–304.

Klerman, Gerald. 1977. "Mental Illness, the Medical Model, and Psychiatry." *The Journal of Medicine and Philosophy* 2(3):220–243.

Klerman, Gerald. 1986. "Historical Perspectives on Contemporary Schools of Psychopathology." Pp. 3–27 in *Contemporary Directions in Psychopathology: Toward the DSM-IV*, edited by T. Millon and G. Klerman. New York: Guilford Press.

———. 1989. "Comment on John Mirowsky and Catherine Ross's 'Psychiatric Diagnosis as Reified Measurement'." *Journal of Health and Social Behavior* 30(March):26–32.

Knorr-Cetina, Karin. 1983. "The Ethnographic Study of Scientific Work: Towards a Constructivist Interpretation of Science." Pp. 115–140 in *Science Observed: Perspectives on the Social Study of Science*, edited by Karin Knorr-Cetina and Michael Mulkay. Beverly Hills: Sage.

Koeske, Randi. 1983. "Lifting the Curse of Menstruation: Toward a Feminist Perspective on the Menstrual Cycle." *Women & Health* 8(2/3):1–16.

Kuhn, Thomas. [1962] 1970. *The Structure of Scientific Revolutions*, Second Edition, Enlarged. Chicago: University of Chicago Press.

Kutchins, Herb, and Stuart Kirk. 1988. "The Future of DSM: Scientific and Professional Issues." *The Harvard Medical School Mental Health Letter* 5(3):4–6.

———. 1989a. "DSM-III-R: The Conflict over New Psychiatric Diagnoses." *Health and Social Work* 14(May):91–101.

———. 1989b. "The Prognosis for Social Work Diagnosis." *Social Casework* 70(May):295–304.

The Lancet. 1994. Editorial. "Molecules and Minds." 343 (March 19):681–682.

Lander, Louise. 1988. *Images of Bleeding*. New York: Orlando Press.

Lark, Susan. 1984. *Premenstrual Syndrome Self Help Book: A Woman's Guide to Feeling Good All Month*. Berkeley: Celestial Arts.

Larson, Magali. 1977. *The Rise of Professionalism*. Berkeley: University of California Press.

Latour, Bruno. 1987. *Science in Action*. Cambridge, MA: Harvard University Press.

———. 1988. *The Pasteurization of France*. Cambridge, MA: Harvard University Press.

Latour, Bruno, and Steve Woolgar. 1979. *Laboratory Life: The Construction of Scientific Facts*. Beverly Hills: Sage.

Law, John. 1987. "Technology and Heterogeneous Engineering: The Case of Portuguese Expansion." Pp. 111–134 in *The Social Construction of Technological Systems*, edited by Wiebe Bijker, Thomas Hughes, and Trevor Pinch. Cambridge, MA: MIT Press.

Laws, Sophie. 1990. *Issues of Blood: The Politics of Menstruation*. London: Macmillan.

Laws, Sophie, Valerie Hey, and Andrea Egan. 1985. *Seeing Red: The Politics of Premenstrual Tension*. London: Hutchinson.

Lehman, Betsy. 1993. "A Little Revision Is Creating a Big Furor." *The Boston Globe*, May 10, 1993:33, 36.

Lehrman, Karen. 1988. "What is PMS?" *Consumers' Research* (February):20–22.

Light, Donald. 1988. "Turf Battles and the Theory of Professional Dominance." *Research in the Sociology of Health Care* 7:203–225.

Lippert, Joan. 1994. "Taking the Edge off P.M.S." *New Woman* March 92–96.

Loring, Marti, and Brian Powell. 1988. "Gender, Race, and DSM-III: A Study of the Objectivity of Psychiatric Diagnostic Behavior." *Journal of Health and Social Behavior* 29(March):1–22.

Lunbeck, Elizabeth. 1994. *The Psychiatric Persuasion: Knowledge, Gender, and Power in Modern America*. Princeton: Princeton University Press.

Mackenzie, Donald. 1981. *Statistics in Britain, 1865–1930: The Social Construction of Scientific Knowledge*. Edinburgh: Edinburgh University Press.

Maddox, John. 1991. "Is Homosexuality Hard Wired?" *Nature* 353:13.

Martin, Brian. 1991. *Scientific Knowledge in Controversy: The Social Dynamics of the Fluoridation Debate*. Albany: State University of New York Press.

Martin, Emily. 1987. *The Woman in the Body: A Cultural Analysis of Reproduction*. Boston: Beacon Press.

Mathis, James. 1992. "Psychiatric Diagnosis: A Continuing Controversy." *The Journal of Medicine and Philosophy* 17:253–261.

McCarthy, Lucille, and Joan Gerring. 1994. "Revising Psychiatry's Charter Document DSM-IV." *Written Communication* 11(2):147–192.

McCrea, Frances. 1983. "The Politics of Menopause: The 'Discovery' of a Deficiency Disease." *Social Problems* 31:111–123.

McGovern, Constance. 1985. *Masters of Madness: Social Origins of the American Psychiatric Profession*. Hanover, NH: University Press of New England.

McMillen, Liz. 1993. "Proposal to Define Premenstrual Syndrome as a Mental Disorder Draws Fire." *The Chronicle of Higher Education* March 31, 1993:A8.

Mickelsen, Lynnell. 1986. "Battle of the couch: Who's Ill?" *The Detroit Free Press*, June 4, 1986:1B–3B.

Millon, Theodore. 1986. "On the Past and Future of the DSM-III: Personal Recollections and Projections." Pp. 29–70 in *Contemporary Directions in Psychopathology: Toward the DSM-IV*, edited by T. Millon and G. Klerman. New York: Guilford Press.

Mirowsky, John and Catherine Ross. 1989. "Psychiatric Diagnosis as Reified Measurement." *Journal of Health and Social Behavior* 30(March):11–25.

Nathan, Peter. 1994. "DSM-IV: Empirical, Accessible, Not Yet Ideal." *Journal of Clinical Psychology* 50:103–110.

National Coalition for Women's Mental Health. 1986. *Research Evidence Does not Support the PMDD Diagnosis (Premenstrual Dysphoric Disorder)*. Paper presented at the debate: "Controversies in the Revision of DSM-III." Annual meeting of the American Psychiatric Association, Washington, D.C., May 1986.

Nazzaro, Ann, and Donald Lombard. 1985. *The PMS Solution*. Minneapolis: Winston Press.

Neff, James, Stephanie McFall, and Timothy Cleaveland. 1987. "Psychiatry and Medicine in the US: Interpreting Trends in Medical Specialty Choice." *Sociology of Health and Illness* 9:45–61.

Nelkin, Dorothy (ed.). 1979. *Controversy: Politics of Technical Decisions*. Second edition. Beverly Hills: Sage.

———. 1982. *The Creation Controversy: Science or Scripture in the Schools*. Boston: Beacon Press.

Nelkin, Dorothy (ed.). 1992. *Controversy: Politics of Technical Decisions*, third edition. Beverly Hills: Sage.

News Bulletin Highlights Issue. 1986. "New DSM Category of PMDD Generates Heated Debate." 7(1):1–2.

New York Times. 1987. "Debated Psychiatric Manual Issued." Tuesday, May 19:C20.

Norris, Ronald, and Colleen Sullivan. 1983. *Premenstrual Syndrome: A Doctor's Proven Program on How to Recognize and Treat PMS*. New York: Berkeley Books.

Olesen, Virginia, and Nancy F. Woods. 1986. *Culture, Society and Menstruation*. Washington: Hemisphere.

Osofsky, Howard, and Susan Blumenthal. 1985. *Premenstrual Syndrome: Current Findings and Future Directions*. Washington, DC: American Psychiatric Association Press.

Parlee, Mary Brown. 1973. "The Premenstrual Syndrome." *Psychological Bulletin* 80:454–465.

———. 1987. "Media Treatment of Premenstrual Syndrome." Pp. 189–205 in *Premenstrual Syndrome: Ethical and Legal Implications in a Biomedical Perspective*, edited by B. E. Ginsburg and B. F. Carter. New York: Plenum.

———. 1992. "On PMS and Psychiatric Abnormality." *Feminism & Psychology* 2(1):105–119.

———. 1993. *"Research on 'Premenstrual Syndrome': Controversies and Consolidation, 1968–1993."* Paper presented at the Society for Social Studies of Science, Annual Meeting, West Lafayette, Indiana, November 21, 1993.

Parsons, Talcott. 1939. "The Professions and Social Structure." *Social Forces* 17:457–467.

Pasnau, Robert. 1986. "Response to the Presidential Address: Health Care Crisis: A Campaign for Action." *American Journal of Psychiatry* 143(8):955–959.

Pasnau, Robert. 1987. "Presidential Address: Psychiatry in Medicine: Medicine in Psychiatry." *American Journal of Psychiatry* 144(8):975–979.

Payer, Lynn, with Ken Gross. 1989. "Hell Week." *Ms.* 17(March):28–31.

Peele, Roger. 1986. "Report of the Speaker-Elect." *American Journal of Psychiatry* 143(10):1348–1453.

People Weekly [Anonymous]. 1994. "Rocky Mountain Low." March 28, 1994:42–43.

Peterson, James, and Gerald Markle. 1980. "Controversies in Science and Technology." Pp. 5–18 in *Science off the Pedestal: Social Perspectives on Science and Technology*, edited by Daryl Chubin and Ellen Chu. Belmont, CA: Wadsworth.

Pickering, Andrew. 1984. *Constructing Quarks: A Sociological History of Particle Physics*. Edinburgh: Edinburgh University Press.

Pinch, Trevor, and Wiebe Bijker. 1987. "The Social Construction of Facts and Artifacts: Or How the Sociology of Science and the Sociology of Technology Might Benefit Each Other." Pp. 17–50 in *The Social Construction of Technological Systems*, edited by Wiebe Bijker, Thomas Hughes, and Trevor Pinch. Cambridge, MA: MIT Press.

Pincus, Harold, Allen Frances, Wendy Davis, Michael First, and Thomas Widiger. 1992. "DSM-IV and New Diagnostic Categories: Holding the Line on Proliferation." *American Journal of Psychiatry* 149:112–117.

Psychiatric News. 1983–1990. The newspaper of the American Psychiatric Association. Articles are cited by date in the text.

Psychiatric Times. 1986. "Science or Politics? DSM-III-R Controversy Grows." III (8):1,17.

Pugliesi, Karen. 1992. "Premenstrual Syndrome: The Medicalization of Emotion Related to Conflict and Chronic Role Strain." *Humbolt Journal of Social Relations* 18(2):131–165.

Reid, Robert. 1986. "Premenstrual Syndrome: A Time for Introspections." *The American Journal of Obstetrics and Gynecology* 155(5):921–926.

Riessman, Catherine Kohler. 1983. "Women and Medicalization: A New Perspective." *Social Policy* 14(1):3–18.

Rittenhouse, Amanda. 1989. *The Emergence of Premenstrual Syndrome: The Social History of a Woman's Health 'Problem'*. Unpublished Ph.D. dissertation, University of California, San Francisco.

Rittenhouse, Amanda. 1991. "The Emergence of Premenstrual Syndrome as a Social Problem." *Social Problems* 38(3):412–425.

Rivera-Tovar, Ana, and Ellen Frank. 1990."Late Luteal Phase Dysphoric Disorder in Young Women." *The American Journal of Psychiatry* 147(12):1634–1636.

Roark, Anne. 1988. "Psychiatric Bible: Old Disorders Given New Labels." *The Los Angeles Times* September 29:24, 28–29.

Robins, Lee and John Helzer. 1986. "Diagnosis and Clinical Assessment: The Current State of Psychiatric Diagnosis." *Annual Review of Psychology* 37:409–32.

Rodin, Mari. 1992. "The Social Construction of Premenstrual Syndrome." *Social Science and Medicine* 35(1):49–56.

Rome, Ester. 1983. *Premenstrual Syndrome (PMS) Examined Through a Feminist Lens*. Boston Women's Health Collective, unpublished manuscript.

Rothman, David. 1971. *The Discovery of the Asylum: Social Order and Disorder in the New Republic*. Boston: Little Brown.

Rovner, Sandy. 1987. "A New Manual for Mental Disorders." *The Washington Post* May 12 (Health):12–13.

Rubinow, David, Peter Roy-Byrne, Christine Hoban, Philip Gold and Robert Post. 1984. American Journal of Psychiatry 141:684–86.

Ruzek, Sheryl. 1978. *The Women's Health Movement: Feminist Alternatives to Medical Control*. New York: Praeger.

———. 1981. "The Women's Self-Help Health Movement." Pp. 563–570 in *The Sociology of Health and Illness: Critical Perspectives*, edited by Peter Conrad and Rochelle Kern. New York: St. Martin's Press.

Sabshin, Melvin. 1986. "Report of the Medical Director." *American Journal of Psychiatry* 143(10):1342–1346.

Schacht, Thomas, and P. E. Nathan. 1977. "But Is It Good for Psychologists?: Appraisal and Status of DSM-III." *American Psychologist* 32:1017–1025.

Schatzman, Leonard, and Anselm Strauss. 1972 [1966]. "A Sociology of Psychiatry: A Perspective and Some Organizing Foci." Pp. 128–144 in *Medical Men and Their Work*, edited by Eliot Friedson and Judith Lorber. Chicago: Aldine/Atherton.

Scheff, Thomas. [1966] 1984. *Being Mentally Ill: A Sociological Theory*, Second Edition. New York: Aldine.

Schmidt, Peter, Lynnett Nieman, Gay Grover, et al. 1991. "Lack of Effect of Induced Menses on Symptoms in Women with Premenstrual Syndrome." *The New England Journal of Medicine* 324(April 25):1174–1179.

Scott, Pam, Evelleen Richards, and Brian Martin. 1990. "Captives of Controversy: The Myth of the Neutral Social Researcher in Contemporary Scientific Controversies." *Science, Technology & Human Values* 15(4):474–494.

Scott, Wilbur. 1990. "PTSD in DSM-III: A Case in the Politics of Diagnosis and Disease." *Social Problems* 37(3):294–310.

Scull, Andrew. 1979. *Museums of Madness: The Social Organization of Insanity in Nineteenth-Century England*. New York: St. Martins Press.

Scully, Diana, and Pauline Bart. 1973. "A Funny Thing Happened on the Way to the

Orifice: Women in Gynecology Textbooks." *American Journal of Sociology* 78 (January):1045–1050.

Seligmann, Jean, with David Gelman 1993. "Is It Sadness or Madness?: Psychiatrists Clash Over How to Classify PMS." *Newsweek* March 15, 1993:66.

Severino, Sally. "Late Luteal Phase Dysphoric Disorder: A Scientific Puzzle." *Medical Hypothesis* 41(3):229–234.

———. 1994. "Commentary: Late Luteal Phase Dysphoric Disorder—Disease or Dis-Ease?" Pp. 213–30 in *Premenstrual Dysphorias: Myths and Realities*, edited by Judith Gold and Sally Severino. Washington, DC: American Psychiatric Association.

Severino, Sally, and Margaret Moline. 1989. *Premenstrual Syndrome: A Clinician's Guide*. New York: The Guilford Press.

Shapin, Steve. 1984. "Pump and Circumstance: Robert Boyle's Literary Technology." *Social Studies of Science* 14:481–520.

Showalter, Elaine. 1985. *The Female Malady: Women, Madness and English Culture, 1830–1980*. New York: Pantheon.

Shuttle, Penelope, and Peter Redgrove. 1978. *The Wise Wound: Eve's Curse and Everywoman*. New York: Richard Marek.

Smith, Harvey. 1954. "Psychiatry: A Social Institution in Process." *Social Forces* 33:310–316.

Smith-Rosenberg, Carroll. 1972. "The Hysterical Woman." *Social Research* 39: 652–678.

Sneed, Sharon, and Joe McIlhaney. 1989. "How to Manage PMS." *Focus on the Family* July:14–16.

Solomon, Alisa. 1993. "Girl Crazy? Psychiatry Tries to Make PMS a Mental Illness." *Village Voice* April 6, 1993:32–33.

Span, Paula. 1993. "Vicious Cycle: The Politics of Periods: After Tomorrow, Many Women May Be Told They're Plain Crazy." *The Washington Post* July 8, 1993:C1–C2.

Spitzer, Robert. 1991. "An Outsider-Insider's Views about Revising the DSMs." *Journal of Abnormal Psychology* 100:294–296.

Spitzer, Robert, and Janet Williams. 1987a. "Introduction" to *Diagnostic and Statistical Manual of Mental Disorders*, Third Edition, Revised. Washington, DC: The American Psychiatric Association.

———. 1987b. "Revising DSM-III: The Process and Major Issues." Chapter 26 in *Diagnosis and Classification in Psychiatry: A Critical Appraisal of DSM-III*, edited by Gary Tischler. Cambridge: Cambridge University Press.

Spitzer, Robert, Janet Williams, and Andrew Skodol. 1980. "DSM-III: The Major Achievements and an Overview." *American Journal of Psychiatry* 137(2): 151–164.

Spitzer, Robert, Sally Severino, Janet Williams, and Barbara Parry. 1989. "Late Luteal Phase Dysphoric Disorder and DSM-III-R." *American Journal of Psychiatry* 146(7):892–897.

Squires, Sally. 1994. "New Guide to Mental Illness: Diagnostic Manual Takes Scientific Approach." *Washington Post* April 12, 1994, Section WH:10.

Star, Susan Leigh. 1988. "Introduction: The Sociology of Science and Technology." *Social Problems* 35(3):197–205.

Star, Susan Leigh, and James Griesemer. 1989. "Institutional Ecology, 'Translations' and Boundary Objects: Amateurs and Professionals in Berkeley's Museum of Vertebrate Zoology, 1907–1939." *Social Studies of Science* 19:387–420.

Starr, Paul. 1982. *The Social Transformation of American Medicine: The Rise of a Sovereign Profession and the Making of Vast Industry.* New York: Basic Books.

Staver, Sari. 1986a. "Diagnostic Disputes: Proposed Changes in Diagnosis Manual Spark Heated Controversies." *American Medical News* June 6:3, 25–28.

———. 1986b. "APA Reaches Compromise on Diagnoses." *American Medical News* July 18:1, 41.

Steiner, Meir, Susanne Steinberg, Donna Stewart, Diana Carter, Charlene Berger, Robert Reid, Douglas Grover, and David Streiner. 1995. "Fluoxetine in the Treatment of Premenstrual Dysphoria." *The New England Journal of Medicine* 332(23):1529–1534.

Strauss, Anselm. 1978. A Social Worlds Perspective. Pp. 119–128 in *Studies in Symbolic Interaction*, vol. 1, edited by Norman Denzin. Greenwich: JAI Press.

Suh, May. 1993. "Severe PMS: Is It Mental Illness or Just Normal Behavior." *Ms.* May/June:90.

Szasz, Thomas. 1970. *The Manufacture of Madness.* New York: Harper & Row.

———. 1974. *The Myth of Mental Illness: Foundations of a Theory of Personal Conduct.* New York: Harper & Row.

Szasz, Thomas. [1963] 1989. *Law, Liberty and Psychiatry.* Syracuse, NY: Syracuse University Press.

Tavris, Carol. 1992. *The Mismeasure of Women.* New York: Simon & Schuster.

Tavris, Carol. 1993. "You Haven't Come Very Far, Baby." *Los Angeles Times*, March 4, 1993:B7.

Taylor, Dena. 1988. *Red Flower: Rethinking Menstruation.* Freedom, CA: The Crossing Press.

Thomas, William I., and Dorothy S. Thomas. 1928. *The Child in America.* New York: Knopf.

Todd, Alexandra. 1989. *Intimate Adversaries: Cultural Conflict between Doctors and Women Patients.* Philadelphia: University of Pennsylvania Press.

Tomes, Nancy. 1990. "Historical Perspectives on Women and Mental Illness." Chapter 6 in *Women, Health and Medicine in America: A Historical Handbook*, edited by Rima D. Apple. New York: Garland.

Ussher, Jane. 1989. *The Psychology of the Female Body.* London: Routledge.

———. 1992. *Women's Madness: Misogyny or Mental Illness?* Amherst: The University of Massachusetts Press.

Vaitukaitis, Judith. 1984. "Premenstrual Syndrome." *New England Journal of Medicine* 311(November 22):1371–1373.

Vigliani, Marguerite. 1988. "PMS: Symptom or Diagnosis." *Journal of the American Medical Women's Association* 43(6):181–182.

Vines, Gail. 1994. "Have Periods, Will Seek Therapy." *New Scientist* 139:1884 (July 31, 1994):12–13.

Vogue. 1985. "Premenstrual Syndrome [reprint of August 1984 *The Harvard Medical School Health Letter*]." June:306–308.

Wade, Carlson. 1984. *Carlson Wade's PMS Book: What You Need to Know.* New Canaan, CT: Keats.

Walker, Lenore. 1986a. "Masochistic Personality Disorder Take Two: A Report from the Front Lines." *FTI Interchange* 4(1):1–2.

———. 1986b. "Memo: Update and Report on Washington, D.C." *Coalition Against Misdiagnosis Newsletter* May 20, 1986.

Washington Post. Editorial. 1991. "'Raging Hormonal Influence.'" June 8, 1991:A20.

Weideger, Paula. 1976. *Menstruation and Menopause: The Physiology and Psychology, the Myth and the Reality*. New York: Knopf.

Widiger, Thomas, Allen Frances, Harold Pincus, and Wendy Davis. 1990. "DSM-IV Literature Reviews: Rationale, Process, and Limitations." *Journal of Psychopathology and Behavioral Assessment* 12(3):189–203.

Williams, Janet. 1986. "DSM-III-R: What's All the Fuss About?" *Hospital and Community Psychiatry* 37(6):549–550.

Williamson, Martha, and Robin Sheets. 1989. *Raging Hormones: The Unofficial PMS Survival Guide*. New York: Doubleday.

Willis, Judith. 1983."Doing Something About 'The Curse.'" *FDA Consumer* 17:11–14.

Wilson, J. Robert, and Elsie Reid Carrington. 1987. *Obstetrics and Gynecology*, 8th edition. St Louis: C. V. Mosby.

Wilson, Mitchell. 1993. "DSM-III and the Transformation of American Psychiatry: A History." *American Journal of Psychiatry* 150:399–410.

Winner, Langdon. 1980. "Do Artifacts Have Politics?" *Daedalus* 109:121–133.

Woods, Nancy. 1987. "Premenstrual Symptoms: Another Look." *Public Health Reports* 102(Jul/Aug):106–112.

Woolgar, Steve. 1988. *Science: The Very Idea*. Chichester, England: Ellis Horwood Limited.

World Health Organization. 1989. *Lexicon of Psychiatric and Mental Health Terms*, Volume I. Geneva: World Health Organization.

Zehr, Stephen. 1990. *Acid Rain as a Social, Political and Scientific Controversy*. Ph.D. dissertation, Indiana University.

Zita, Jacquelyn. 1988. "The Premenstrual Syndrome 'Dis-easing' the Female Cycle." *Hypatia* 3(1):77–99.

Zola, Irving Kenneth. 1972. "Medicine as an Institution of Social Control." *Sociological Review* 20:487–504.

Index